M O S B Y' S

Emergency
Nursing
Review

M O S B Y' S

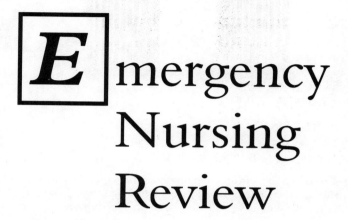

Emergency
Nursing
Review

Reneé Semonin Holleran,
RN, PhD, CEN, CCRN
Chief Flight Nurse, University Air Care,
University of Cincinnati Hospital,
Cincinnati, Ohio

Illustrated

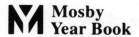
Mosby
Year Book

St. Louis   Baltimore   Boston   Chicago   London   Philadelphia   Sydney   Toronto

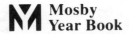

Mosby Year Book

Dedicated to Publishing Excellence

Executive Editor: Don Ladig
Managing Editor: Robin Carter
Editorial Assistant: Ann Winston
Project Manager: Gayle May Morris
Production Editor: Judith Bange
Book Design: Jeanne Wolfgeher

Printed in the United States of America

Mosby–Year Book, Inc., 11830 Westline Industrial Drive, St. Louis, MO 63146

Library of Congress Cataloging-in-Publication Data

Holleran, Reneé Semonin.
   Mosby's emergency nursing review / Reneé Semonin Holleran.
      p.   cm.
   Includes bibliographical references and index.
   ISBN 0-8016-2462-2
      1. Emergency nursing—Examinations, questions, etc.   I. Title.
   II. Title: Emergency nursing review.
      [DNLM: 1. Critical care—examination questions. 2. Emergencies—examination questions. 3. Emergency Service, Hospital—examination questions. 4. Nursing—examination questons. WY 18 H737m]
RT120.E4H65   1992
610.73´61´076—dc20
DNLM/DLC
for Library of Congress   91–14164
                                                                                    CIP

GW/DC   9   8   7   6   5   4   3   2   1

Contributors

Terry Matthew Foster, RN, CEN, CCRN

Clinical Director, Nursing Administration, Mercy Hospital, Cincinnati, Ohio;
Staff Nurse, Emergency Department, St. Elizabeth Medical Center, Covington, Kentucky

Susan Mills, RN, CEN

Staff Nurse, Emergency Department, University Hospital, Cincinnati, Ohio;
Staff Nurse, Emergency Department, St. Elizabeth Medical Center, Covington, Kentucky

Mary Ann Niehaus, RN, MSN, CEN, REMT-P

Head Nurse, Emergency Department, St. Francis/St. George Hospital, Cincinnati, Ohio

T. Jane Swaim, RN, MS

Assistant Administrator, Emergency, Trauma, Critical Care, Neuroscience, University Hospital, Cincinnati, Ohio

Consultants

Geri Dees, RN, MN
Clinical Specialist, Trauma and Emergency Nursing, University of California at Los Angeles, Los Angeles, California

Lynn Eastes, RN, MS
Trauma Coordinator, Oregon Health Sciences University, Portland, Oregon

Pamela Frankel, RN, MS
Trauma Coordinator, Oregon Health Sciences University, Portland, Oregon

Susan Fraser, RN, MSN, CEN
Staff Nurse, Emergency Services, University of Alabama Hospital, Birmingham, Alabama

Catherine Hall, RN, MS
Trauma Nurse Coordinator, Trauma Program, Miami Valley Hospital, Dayton, Ohio

Sue Moore, RN, MS, CCRN, CEN
Clinical Specialist, Emergency Services, Washoe Medical Center, Reno, Nevada

Gail Mornhinweg, RN, PhD
Associate Professor, School of Nursing, University of Louisville, Louisville, Kentucky

George O. Pankiw, RN, EMT-P
Chief Flight Nurse, Life Force, Erlanger Medical Center, Chattanooga, Tennessee

Jacquelyn Reid, BSN, MA, EdD
Associate Professor, School of Nursing, University of Louisville, Louisville, Kentucky

Darlene Schelper, RN, MSN, CEN
Clinical Educator, Emergency Services, Hershey Medical Center, Hershey, Pennsylvania

Patricia Southard, RN, JD, CEN
Program Director, Trauma, Oregon Health Sciences University, Portland, Oregon

Joe E. Taylor, RN, PhD, CEN, CNAA, NREMT-P
Vice-President, South Central Regional Medical Center, Laurel, Mississippi

This book is dedicated first to my family, Micke, Erin, Sara, and my mother. Second, I dedicate this book to all of us who practice emergency nursing. As I have come to find, nursing is a way of life.

Foreword

Taking the Certified Emergency Nurse Examination

The emergency nursing certification examination was first offered in July 1980 by the Board of Certification for Emergency Nursing. The registered nurse who passes this test is designated as a certified emergency nurse, or CEN. Certification is a process whereby qualifications are validated and knowledge for practice in a defined functional or clinical area of nursing is measured. The purpose of the CEN examination is to provide a method of measuring the attainment and application of emergency nursing at a competency level.

The CEN examination is divided into the following areas of nursing practice:

Assessment	30.5%
Analysis/nursing diagnosis	15.0%
Planning/intervention	30.0%
Evaluation	14.5%
Professional issues	10.0%
	100.0% (TOTAL)

The exam contains a maximum of 250 multiple-choice questions with a total testing time of 4 hours.

There are several ways to prepare for taking the CEN examination. The following are some test-taking strategies to help you increase your test-taking skills and improve your test scores.

1. Obtain a *CEN Examination Handbook* as soon as possible. This will contain the necessary information about the CEN examination (dates, deadlines, application forms, fees, etc.). You are responsible for knowing its content. After reading this handbook, you will know exactly what is expected of you. Having this knowledge will increase your confidence.

Single copies of the *CEN Examination Handbook* and applications may be obtained from:

Board of Certification for Emergency Nursing
230 East Ohio Street, Suite 600
Chicago, IL 60611-3297
(312) 649-0297

Bulk quantitites (two or more) of the handbook and applications may be obtained from:
Certification Examination for Emergency Nurses
American College Testing (82)
P.O. Box 168
Iowa City, IA 52243
(319) 337-1283

Members of the Emergency Nurses Association receive a discount on the CEN examination. For an ENA membership application, contact:
Emergency Nurses Association
Membership Services Division
230 East Ohio Street, Suite 600
Chicago, IL 60611-3297
(312) 649-0297

2. Prepare for the examination a few months before the test date. Set aside an hour or two a few days each week to review the major content areas of the exam. Review *Mosby's Emergency Nursing Review* and/or the Emergency Nursing Core Curriculum of the ENA thoroughly. Carefully review the questions in this book until you are able to answer most of them correctly.

Consider a CEN examination review course, and ask yourself the following questions: Will this course actually help me to pass the exam? Who are the faculty? Are the faculty members CENs? What are the objectives of the course? Is the course accredited? Most of these courses help you to identify *your* learning needs. They are not a substitute for studying.

Talk to your nursing colleagues who are CENs. Ask what worked for them in preparing for the exam. Do they have any other suggestions?

Review advanced cardiac life support (ACLS) and basic life support (BLS) courses or become recertified. Many questions on the examination come directly from these standards of care. Therefore it is important that you know them.

Concentrate on those areas you have identified as areas of weakness. If, for example, your knowledge or understanding of arterial blood gases (ABGs) is lacking, concentrate on this subject for a few days. Read a chapter on respiratory physiology from a pathophysiology text. Copy and read journal articles on ABGs. Practice ABG interpretation on each of your patients who have ABGs drawn. Discuss your findings with another nurse or physician. Applying principles to the clinical setting is the best way for most nurses to learn. Remember, the key here is to study, but also to keep your studying clinically focused.

It may help to keep your review materials handy, especially at work, to review during those occasional slower times in the emergency department. You might read appropriate emergency care journals to break the studying monotony and increase your knowledge base. It may also help to keep a simple log on how much time you spend reviewing (even if it is only 10 minutes between appointments). After a while you may be surprised to see how much unscheduled time you have accumulated in studying for this exam. This will help boost your self-confidence.

One more thing about spending time preparing for the CEN examination: since the exam is based on current emergency nursing practice, think about how many hours you have worked in the emergency department. Full-time employment works out to be about 2080 hours per year; part-time employment is about 1040 hours per year. The *best* way to be prepared for this exam is to have at least 2 years of current emergency nursing experience . . . so you may have already spent thousands of hours in preparation for this exam. You may know more than you think, but, nonetheless, be prepared.

If you have not tested well in the past, or if you have not taken a test in several years, consider taking the practice exams in other review books (e.g., RN state board review books), as well as answering the review questions in this book. Familiarizing yourself with the format of multiple-choice questions before you take the exam will make taking the test less daunting.

3. The night before the test, be sure to get a good night's sleep. Avoid any alcohol or drugs to help you sleep. They will affect your performance the following day. Eat a good but light breakfast to "feed your brain" as well as your stomach.

4. As you begin to take the test, remember to relax. Anxiety will prevent you from doing a good job. Do not let brief and needless anxiety affect your knowledge of emergency nursing. Your skills are tested everyday with human lives; sitting down to take an exam is the easy part of an emergency nurse's job.

5. Some things to keep in mind when reading and answering test questions:

During the exam, periodically check to make sure you are answering the questions in the proper space. This could prevent a serious error that could cause several answers to be incorrect.

Remember a cardinal rule for test taking: always keep the first answer you choose. Do not go back and change an answer unless you are certain the new one is correct.

Do not overlook key words such as *early, late, except, not, immediate,* or *nursing action.*

There is usually no pattern to the answers on a test. Do not select *B* simply because you have not used a *B* in the last 10 answers.

Beware of answer choices that contain qualifiers such as *always, never, all,* or *every.* These are blanket terms, and we know that in nursing nothing is ever 100% certain. Answers that contain these words can usually — but not always — be considered false.

What if you come to a question that confuses you? First of all, it cannot be overemphasized how clinically oriented this examination is. Imagine yourself in that particular clinical situation. What would you do? You may be surprised at how automatically some answers to confusing questions will come to you if you put yourself in the clinical setting. Plus, keep in mind, who is better at sorting out confusion than an emergency nurse?

If you come to a question for which you have no idea what the answer is, return to it later. Perhaps another question on the test may give you a clue to the correct answer. Narrow your choices to a question by eliminating obviously wrong answers. Also, there is no penalty for guessing, so answering every question will increase your chances of getting a high score.

Finally, we wish you well. It is a big commitment to work toward becoming a CEN. Congratulations on putting forth the effort. We hope that these suggestions will make taking the exam a more positive experience. The time that you have put into studying will pay off. Good luck.

Terry Matthew Foster

Preface

EMERGENCY NURSING AND CERTIFICATION

The practice of emergency nursing requires a *unique* body of knowledge. The emergency nurse has to be a specialist who practices in complex situations requiring a great deal of knowledge about a lot of things. Emergency nurses experience many types of patient care situations within their practice. The emergency nurse essentially must be prepared for anything.

In 1991 the Emergency Nurses Association (ENA) completed the revision of the *Standards of Emergency Nursing Practice.*[1] Comprehensive Standard 12 states that "emergency nurses shall be competent and current—adhering to established standards of practice. Safe and effective emergency nursing practice depends on the retention and application of a specific body of knowledge and skills that are dynamic over time." Continuing education and the achievement of certification in emergency nursing are two ways the emergency nurse can prepare for and continue providing safe and effective emergency nursing care.

The practice of emergency nursing is a specialty component of the nursing profession. As professionals, emergency nurses have an obligation to the people they care for to define what their distinctive body of knowledge is. Once this knowledge has been identified, emergency nurses need to be accountable for what they profess.[2] Accountability is achieved through the adoption of standards of practice, a code of ethics, research, and certification.[2]

Two specific goals of certification include assuring consumer access to care and consumer and provider protection.[2] Certification can provide consumer access to care by demonstrating that nurses have gained a certain body of knowledge to practice in a specific role. Some examples of this type of certification include that for nurse-midwives and that for pediatric nurse practitioners.

Certification can provide protection for both the consumer and the provider of nursing care by allowing only qualified individuals to be involved in specialized nursing practice. For example, the practice of emergency nursing requires a distinctive knowledge base. When emergency nurses have achieved the Certification in Emergency Nursing (CEN), they have demonstrated their knowledge of emergency nursing.

THE NURSING PROCESS

The certification exam given by the Board of Certification for Emergency Nursing is based on the nursing process.[3] The nursing process is a problem-solving process that nurses use to provide care for patients. The components of the nursing process include assessment (data collection), analysis (nursing diagnosis), intervention (independent and collaborative), and evaluation.[4]

Assessment

Comprehensive Standard 2 from the *Standards of Emergency Nursing Practice* states that "emergency nurses shall initiate accurate and ongoing assessment of physical and psychosocial problems with the emergency care system."[1] When collecting data about the patient, the emergency nurse collects both subjective and objective information. Patient assessment in the emergency department generally is episodic and related to the reason why the patient has come to the emergency department. Current and past medical history, social support, and past emergency department experiences can provide key clues in identifying the health needs of the emergency department patient.[2,3]

Analysis

The analysis component of the nursing process summarizes the data collected during the patient assessment. Based on this summary, the emergency nurse determines the patient's potential or actual health problems.[3] Comprehensive Standard 3 from the *Standards of Emergency Nursing Practice* states that "the systematic process of patient assessment and data analysis is reflected in appropriate nursing diagnosis and decision making."[1]

Nursing diagnoses are used as a means of identifying the patient's potential or actual health care problems and as a framework on which emergency nurses can base their interventions and evaluate the effectiveness of these interventions. The North American Nursing Diagnosis Association (NANDA) has identified over 100 different nursing diagnoses. Research continues on the development of even more. Several sources for nursing diagnoses include their definitions, defining characteristics, and related findings. Useful texts containing nursing diagnoses and their application to clinical nursing practice are included in several of the References and/or Additional Readings sections, which are located at the end of each chapter.

Intervention

Interventions are specific nursing and collaborative measures taken to meet the emergency department patient's potential or actual health care needs. Comprehensive Standard 5 from the *Standards of Emergency Nursing Practice* states that "emergency nurses shall implement a plan of care based on assessment data, nursing and medical diagnosis."[1]

Emergency nursing interventions can be either independent or collaborative. Independent emergency nursing interventions are based on specific practice parameters established by the profession of nursing.[1] Collaborative interventions include care provided by other health care personnel, along with the emergency nurse, including physicians, social workers, and prehospital care personnel.

Evaluation

The final component of the nursing process is evaluation. The function of evaluation is to examine whether the interventions performed by the emergency nurse—either independently or collaboratively—have been effective. Comprehensive Standard 6 from the *Standards of Emergency Nursing Practice* states that "evaluation of emergency care must be based on patient care standards, observable patient outcomes, and patient goals."[1]

The effectiveness of independent and collaborative emergency nursing care can be evaluated using several methods. These include attainment of patient goals, quality assurance plans, chart audits, and direct observation of the patient's response to interventions.[1]

HOW TO USE THIS BOOK

The immense scope of emergency nursing practice makes it difficult for any one text to contain all aspects of emergency nursing. In addition, it is difficult for any one text, journal, or periodical to keep abreast of all the nursing, medical, and societal changes that occur of which the emergency nurse must be aware. Perhaps this is one of the reasons why many of us practice in the emergency department. There is always some new challenge awaiting us.

The purpose of this book is to provide the emergency nurse with a text that contains many of the elements of emergency nursing in question form. Each chapter begins with a Review Outline. This outline contains suggested material that may be helpful to the emergency nurse for review. The outline is followed by an Introduction, which is a brief discussion of the topic. This is followed by a series of Review Questions in case study or miscellaneous format. There are 565 questions in all. The questions are multiple choice and in most cases include four options (*A* through *D*); we suggest you indicate your answer by filling in the oval shape (0) that precedes each option and that you refer to the answers at the end of the chapter only after you have completed all questions.

The questions in the book are based on the nursing process, and the answers indicate whether the question relates to nursing assessment, analysis (nursing diagnosis), intervention, or evaluation. In some cases the correct answers are referenced; and References and/or Additional Readings are included at the end of each chapter.

• • •

The chapters contained in the book are based on the Emergency Nursing Core Curriculum.[5] Included in the book are such fundamentals of emergency nursing as abdominal emergencies, environmental emergencies, organ procurement, and patient care management. Since emergency nurses are both female and male, the exclusive use of the pronouns *his, her, he,* or *she* has been avoided.

This book was written by practicing emergency nurses. We all practice in various emergency departments, including community and inner-city facilities. We hope it will help all of you in reviewing the knowledge base of emergency nursing. We also hope it reflects how proud we are to be emergency nurses, and we welcome your comments for future editions.

Renee Semonin Holleran

REFERENCES

1. Emergency Nurses Association (ENA): *Standards of emergency nursing practice*, ed 2, St Louis, 1991, Mosby–Year Book.
2. Bulechek GM, Maas ML: Nursing certification: a matter for the professional organization. In McCloskey JC, Grace HK, editors: *Current issues in nursing*, ed 3, St Louis, 1990, Mosby–Year Book.
3. Kidd P: Defining nursing process categories in the emergency nursing certification examination, *JEN* 16:78A-80A, 1990.
4. McFarland GK, McFarlane EA: *Nursing diagnosis and intervention: planning for patient care,* St Louis, 1989, Mosby–Year Book.
5. Rea R et al: *Emergency nursing core curriculum,* ed 3, Philadelphia, 1987, WB Saunders.

Brief Contents

Detailed Contents

MOSBY'S

Emergency Nursing Review

Chapter 1 _____

Abdominal Emergencies

REVIEW OUTLINE

I. Anatomy and physiology
    A. Abdominal organs
        1. Spleen
        2. Liver
        3. Stomach
        4. Small intestine
        5. Large intestine
        6. Umbilicus
        7. Pancreas
        8. Gallbladder
        9. Appendix
       10. Mesentery
       11. Descending aorta
       12. Inferior vena cava
       13. Iliac artery
       14. Renal artery
    B. Physiology
        1. Digestion
        2. Absorption
        3. Elimination
        4. Bile production and excretion
        5. Liver function
        6. Insulin production and use
        7. Red blood cell and white blood cell production and destruction
II. Abdominal assessment
    A. History
        1. Pain

a. Location
b. Quality
c. Severity
d. Radiation
e. Timing
f. Provocative, palliative

2. Vomiting
   a. Onset
   b. Frequency
   c. Duration
   d. Amount
   e. Color, consistency

3. Other associated symptoms
   a. Bleeding
   b. Change in bowel habit
   c. Change in appetite
   d. Recent weight change
   e. Fever, chills

4. Mechanism of injury
   a. Blunt
   b. Penetrating

5. Pertinent medical history
   a. Current or chronic diseases
   b. Past surgeries
   c. Current medications
      (1) Prescribed
      (2) Over-the-counter
      (3) Illicit
   d. Allergies
   e. Alcohol use
   f. Recent foreign travel

B. Physical examination
   1. Overview
      a. Positioning
      b. Facial expression
      c. Skin color, temperature, moisture
   2. Vital signs
   3. Inspection
      a. Abdominal wall movement
      b. Presence of scars
      c. Distention, ascites

        d. Pulsatile mass

        e. Signs of trauma

    4. Auscultation

        a. Bowel sounds

           (1) Present or absent

           (2) Character

        b. Bruits

    5. Palpation

        a. Tenderness

        b. Rigidity, guarding

        c. Masses

        d. Rebound tenderness

  C. Diagnostic studies or procedures

    1. Complete blood cell count (CBC) with differential

    2. Electrolytes, blood urea nitrogen (BUN), blood sugar (BS) or glucose, creatinine

    3. Amylase

    4. Beta human chorionic gonadotropin (BHCG)

    5. Liver profile

    6. Urinalysis

    7. Cultures

    8. Stool for ova, parasites

    9. Test for presence of blood in feces, vomit, and/or nasogastric drainage

   10. Upright chest x-ray film

   11. Upright, left lateral decubitus, flat abdominal x-ray films

   12. Contrast studies

   13. Scanning

   14. Ultrasound

   15. Gastroscopy, endoscopy, sigmoidoscopy

   16. Peritoneal lavage

   17. Local wound exploration

III. Related nursing diagnoses

  A. Anxiety

  B. Constipation

  C. Coping, ineffective individual

  D. Diarrhea

  E. Fear

  F. Fluid volume deficit (actual or potential)

  G. Gas exchange, impaired

  H. Hyperthermia

I. Knowledge deficit
J. Infection, potential for
K. Nutrition, altered: less than body requirements
L. Pain
M. Tissue perfusion, altered (gastrointestinal, renal)
IV. Collaborative care of the patient with an abdominal emergency
    A. Oxygen therapy
    B. Monitoring
        1. Vital signs
        2. Cardiac monitoring
        3. Intake and output
    C. Intravenous fluids
    D. Blood administration
    E. Gastric decompression
    F. Identification and control of bleeding
        1. Cool saline lavage
        2. Balloon tamponade
    G. Autotransfusion
        1. Autotransfusor
        2. Pneumatic antishock garment (PASG)
    H. Peritoneal lavage
    I. Pharmacological intervention
        1. Analgesics
        2. Antibiotics
        3. Antiemetics
        4. Antispasmotics, anticholinergics
        5. Histamine receptor antagonists
        6. Antacids
    J. Emotional support
    K. Patient/family teaching
V. Specific abdominal emergencies
    A. Inflammatory diseases
        1. Esophagitis
        2. Gastritis
        3. Gastroenteritis
        4. Diverticulitis
        5. Pancreatitis
        6. Appendicitis
        7. Hepatitis
        8. Cholecystitis

    B. Intestinal obstruction, intussusception
    C. Esophageal varices
    D. Gastric or duodenal ulcer
    E. Abdominal aortic aneurysm
    F. Abdominal trauma
       1. Penetrating
          a. Gunshot wounds
          b. Stab wounds
       2. Blunt
          a. Organ contusion
          b. Organ laceration
          c. Organ rupture

INTRODUCTION

Abdominal complaints account for a significant percentage of patient complaints handled by the emergency nurse. They may be the manifestation of an acute process or a chronic, long-standing problem. Pain may arise from one of many systems located in the abdomen: the gastrointestinal, genitourinary, and gynecological systems take up most of the organ space. In addition, the vascular and musculoskeletal systems may be involved. Likewise, trauma to the abdomen may involve any of these systems.

The abdominal cavity is large and located anteriorly, making it more susceptible to both blunt and penetrating injury. As the diaphragm rises with expiration, the abdominal cavity size increases, and injury to its contents may occur with a lower chest injury. Blunt trauma results in a force being diffused throughout the abdomen. Penetrating injury, caused by any object that penetrates the abdominal wall, usually a bullet, knife, or some type of missile, injures anything in its path.[1] When solid organs of the abdomen, such as the liver, spleen, and kidneys, are injured, significant bleeding results. When hollow organs, such as the stomach and intestines, are damaged, their contents spill, causing massive irritation and infection.

Abdominal pain may be classified according to type. Visceral pain, so named because it is caused by the stretching of a hollow viscus, is characterized by diffuse crampy pain varying in intensity. Many inflammatory conditions, such as appendicitis, cholecystitis, pancreatitis, and intestinal obstruction, present with visceral pain. The second type, somatic or parietal pain, is a result of bacterial or chemical irritation of nerve fibers. This type of pain is sharp in nature and localized. The patient suffering from somatic pain characteristically assumes the fetal position, either on the side or supine with knees flexed, attempting to prevent any movement that will result in increased pain. The third type of abdominal pain, referred pain, is felt some distance from the source.[2] A classic example of referred pain is seen in renal colic when the pain is located in the groin and external genitalia.

Initial nursing care of the patient with an abdominal emergency is based on subjective and objective assessment. A general overview of the patient, including the position he or she assumes, facial expression, and skin color, temperature, and moisture, may give an indication as to the type and severity of pain. Vital signs give important baseline information.

A subjective assessment, or history, using the PQRST mnemonic (provocation, quality, radiation, severity, timing), is a useful tool in evaluating the patient with an abdominal complaint. Associated signs and symptoms assist in determining which system or systems need further evaluation.

Recognizing abdominal trauma is vital to patient management but is sometimes difficult. The mechanism of injury must be carefully assessed to determine abdominal involvement. In multiple trauma (i.e., trauma involving two or more body systems), abdominal injury is assumed until it has been ruled out. The goal of emergency care in abdominal trauma is to determine whether the patient requires surgery and not to isolate specific injuries.

General management of the patient with an abdominal emergency is determined by evaluation of the ABCs (airway, breathing, circulation) and the initial assessment. Intravenous access for laboratory studies, fluids, and medications is indicated. Other laboratory specimens, such as urine and peritoneal lavage fluid, may be needed. Gastric decompression and bladder catheterization are frequent interventions. Pain management through nursing comfort measures until, and in addition to, pharmacological intervention is important. Infection prevention and/or treatment is indicated. Finally, preparation for admission or discharge involves patient and family teaching and, at discharge, follow-up instructions.[3]

REVIEW QUESTIONS
Gastritis

A 28-year-old woman comes to the emergency department with epigastric pain and vomiting. She is alert, appears uncomfortable, is tearful, and vomits while in triage. Her vital signs are blood pressure, 110/78; pulse, 82; respiratory rate, 20; and temperature, 98.2° F.

1. A part of her history that may be most contributory to her problem is:
   0   A. Her past medical history

   0 B. Any frequency, urgency, or dysuria
   0 C. Her dietary and/or alcohol intake prior to the onset of pain
   0 D. Any recent strenuous activity

2. When the patient describes her vomitus as containing some blood, a simple diagnostic study for the nurse to perform would be a:
   0 A. Stool examination for occult blood
   0 B. Gastric lavage
   0 C. CBC
   0 D. Dipstick or guiac test of current vomitus

3. After an evaluation the physician prescribes prochlorperazine, 10 mg IM. The nurse recognizes the appropriateness of this drug because of its:
   0 A. Antiemetic effect
   0 B. Hypnotic effect
   0 C. Pain-relieving effect
   0 D. Antianxiety effect

4. Based on this patient's persistent vomiting, the appropriate nursing diagnosis is:
   0 A. Injury, potential for
   0 B. Fluid volume deficit
   0 C. Anxiety
   0 D. Nutrition, altered

5. All of the following would assist the emergency nurse in evaluating this patient in terms of adequate fluid volume *except*:
   0 A. Intake and output adequate and approximated
   0 B. Sodium and potassium levels normal
   0 C. Urine specific gravity not significantly increased
   0 D. No complaints of pain or discomfort

Appendicitis

A 5-year-old boy with a 2-day history of abdominal pain and vomiting is referred to the emergency department by his private physician. He is alert and lying quietly. His vital signs are blood pressure, 92/64; pulse, 118; respiratory rate, 24; and temperature, 101.2° F.

6. On careful assessment of this patient's abdomen, the emergency nurse would expect to find:
   0 A. Right lower quadrant (RLQ) tenderness with rebound

0   B. Hyperactive bowel sounds
0   C. Right upper quadrant (RUQ) tenderness radiating to the back
0   D. A pulsatile mass

7. Prompt medical diagnosis and appropriate surgical intervention are necessary in this case to avoid significant complications as reflected by the
   following diagnosis:
   0   A. Fluid volume deficit
   0   B. Pain
   0   C. Infection, potential for
   0   D. Mobility, impaired physical

8. The most useful nursing measure to be taken in order to allay anxiety
   in this patient would be to:
   0   A. Maintain a calm, efficient manner
   0   B. Explain procedures in simple terms
   0   C. Divert the child's attention with a book or toy
   0   D. Have the parent remain with the child

9. The physician orders an IV infusion of dextrose in saline. After establishing the IV infusion, the nurse notes that the child has become restless and
   is crying because of pain. An appropriate initial response would be to:
   0   A. Recheck vital signs, including temperature
   0   B. Ask the physician for an order for sedation
   0   C. Ask the child if he wants a coloring book
   0   D. Attempt repositioning

10. As part of the preparation for surgery, the physician orders cefazolin, 500
    mg IV. The nurse dilutes this in 50 ml of normal saline (NS) and hangs
    it as a piggyback to the present IV infusion in order to prevent which of
    the following complications?
    0   A. Cardiac dysrhythmia
    0   B. Phlebitis at the IV site
    0   C. Nausea and vomiting
    0   D. Dizziness

Pancreatitis

*A 64-year-old woman is brought to the emergency department by the rescue squad.
She complaints of severe upper abdominal pain. She is pale and somewhat diaphoretic.
Her vital signs are blood pressure, 142/72; pulse, 108; respiratory rate, 20; and tem-
perature, 98.1° F.*

11. Initial measures to be taken by the emergency nurse on receiving this patient include all of the following *except*:
    - 0   A. Performing a 12-lead ECG
    - 0   B. Attaching a cardiac monitor
    - 0   C. Identifying unlabeled medications the patient has with her
    - 0   D. Establishing IV access

12. The part of this patient's history that is most contributory to establishing a diagnosis of pancreatitis is:
    - 0   A. Her allergy to sulfa
    - 0   B. Her past mastectomy for cancer
    - 0   C. The fact that she is currently taking antihypertensives
    - 0   D. Her past history of gallstones

13. A recheck of the patient's vital signs reveals a blood pressure of 106/60, a pulse of 122, and a respiratory rate of 24. The skin remains cool and damp. The nursing diagnosis that most accurately reflects this patient's condition is:
    - 0   A. Fluid volume deficit
    - 0   B. Cardiac output, decreased
    - 0   C. Infection, potential for
    - 0   D. Gas exchange, impaired

14. Vigorous fluid resuscitation with balanced electrolyte solution is instituted. A positive response to this therapy would be indicated by all of the following *except*:
    - 0   A. Blood pressure stabilization
    - 0   B. Rales appearing in both bases
    - 0   C. The skin becoming warm and dry
    - 0   D. Increased urine output

15. The diagnosis of acute pancreatitis is confirmed by:
    - 0   A. A markedly elevated amylase level
    - 0   B. An elevated WBC count
    - 0   C. Air-fluid levels on an abdominal x-ray film
    - 0   D. A guaiac-negative emesis and stool

Abdominal Aortic Aneurysm

A 76-year-old man with a sudden onset of severe back and abdominal pain is brought to the emergency department by the rescue squad. His past medical history includes a stroke 2 years ago. He is currently taking antihypertensives. He appears acutely un-

comfortable and is slightly diaphoretic. His vital signs are blood pressure, 124/70;
pulse, 128; respiratory rate, 20; and temperature, 97.7° F.

16. Based on this patient's presentation, which system should the nurse be
    most concerned about in the assessment?
    0   A. Genitourinary system
    0   B. Gastrointestinal system
    0   C. Cardiovascular system
    0   D. Respiratory system

17. The patient's description of his pain alerts the nurse to the severity and
    significance of his condition when he refers to it as:
    0   A. Stabbing
    0   B. Sharp, tearing
    0   C. Dull pressure
    0   D. Crushing

18. The nurse's goal in caring for this patient is to:
    0   A. Provide an environment with diminished stimuli
    0   B. Work toward pain control using both general comfort measures
          and prescribed pharmacological agents
    0   C. Assist in diagnostic studies
    0   D. Prepare the patient for surgery as quickly as possible

19. This patient's primary nursing diagnosis is:
    0   A. Tissue perfusion, altered
    0   B. Pain
    0   C. Infection, potential for
    0   D. Fluid volume deficit

20. The accepted criteria for stabilization in patients with an abdominal
    aortic aneurysm is:
    0   A. A systolic pressure of 90 to 100 mm Hg
    0   B. A hemoglobin of 10 or greater
    0   C. Pain control
    0   D. The absence of cardiac dysrhythmias

Esophageal Varices

A 47-year-old man comes to the emergency department complaining of vomiting blood
for the past several hours. He denies any pain at the present. He is somewhat lethargic

but oriented, slightly jaundiced, warm, and dry, and he smells of alcohol. His vital signs are blood pressure, 146/98; pulse, 98; respiratory rate, 20; and temperature, 98.3° F. As the emergency nurse is interviewing him, he vomits 200 ml of bright red blood.

21. Useful information derived from this patient's past medical history includes all of the following *except* his:
  0 A. Past episodes of upper GI bleeding
  0 B. Past treatment for hypertension
  0 C. Long-term heavy alcohol intake
  0 D. Known liver disease

22. Bleeding from esophageal varices usually stems from:
  0 A. An esophageal perforation
  0 B. An esophageal fistula
  0 C. Pulmonary hypertension
  0 D. Portal hypertension

23. Based on this patient's presentation, the nurse identifies his most urgent nursing diagnosis as:
  0 A. Airway clearance, ineffective
  0 B. Infection, potential for
  0 C. Injury, potential for
  0 D. Nutrition, altered (potential for)

24. Gastric decompression and lavage for this patient would be best accomplished with the use of a:
  0 A. Salem gastric tube
  0 B. Levine gastric tube
  0 C. Blakemore tube
  0 D. Miller-Abbott tube

• • •

25. Nursing interventions for the patient who has a Blakemore tube in place include all of the following *except*:
  0 A. Deflating the esophageal balloon every 8 hours to avoid necrosis
  0 B. Monitoring the patient closely for signs of airway obstruction
  0 C. Keeping equipment at the bedside in case the balloons must be deflated rapidly
  0 D. Carefully reinserting the tube if the balloons accidentally deflate

26. For which of the following laboratory studies would one expect to get an order for vitamin K?
    0   A. Elevated bleeding time
    0   B. Elevated liver enzyme level
    0   C. Elevated BUN
    0   D. Decreased bleeding time

Abdominal Trauma

A 24-year-old woman is brought to the emergency department by the rescue squad, who say she was seen by bystanders to have fallen out of her car. She mumbled something to one of them about being assaulted by her boyfriend earlier that day. She is well-known in the neighborhood as a heavy "crack" user. She is warm, dry, and minimally responsive to painful stimuli. She has no audible blood pressure; her pulse is 150; and her respiratory rate is 48 with poor ventilatory effort.

27. The nurse's first intervention is to:
    0   A. Establish IV access for blood samples and a fluid bolus
    0   B. Attempt to obtain a blood pressure reading via Doppler
    0   C. Assure an open airway and assist ventilations with bag breathing
    0   D. Attach monitor electrodes to determine cardiac rhythm

28. Based on the information given by the EMS personnel, the nurse suspects the underlying cause of this patient's compromised vital signs to be:
    0   A. A head injury resulting from the fall from the car
    0   B. Blunt chest/abdominal trauma resulting from the earlier assault
    0   C. A cocaine overdose
    0   D. Data are insufficient to draw any conclusion at this time

29. The nursing diagnosis that best reflects this patient's initial presentation is:
    0   A. Breathing pattern, ineffective
    0   B. Fluid volume deficit
    0   C. Injury, potential for
    0   D. Pain

30. The physician prepares to perform a peritoneal lavage. The nurse's role in this procedure is:
    0   A. Insertion of a Foley catheter after lavage begins
    0   B. Insertion of a gastric tube after lavage begins

    0   C. Monitoring of cardiac rhythm during the procedure

    0   D. Insertion of a Foley catheter prior to the procedure

31. The lavage returns are frankly bloody. The nurse recognizes that the next function will be:

    0   A. Preparing the patient for an abdominal computed tomography (CT) scan

    0   B. Transferring the patient to a ready operating room

    0   C. Sending lavage fluid to the laboratory for analysis

    0   D. Taking vital signs while the physician is rechecking the position of the lavage catheter

ANSWERS

1. **C. Assessment.** Dietary indiscretions, such as eating too much or too rapidly, or eating food that is irritating to the stomach because of excessive seasoning, are frequent causes of gastritis. Other contributing factors include use of alcohol, tobacco, salicylates, steroids, nonsteroidal antiinflammatory agents, and emotional stress.[4]

2. **D. Assessment.** Any vomiting that occurs during the course of the evaluation of a patient with abdominal pain should be routinely checked for occult blood. A positive finding may be an indication for more invasive procedures, such as gastric lavage or gastroscopy, to rule out ulcer disease.

3. **A. Intervention.** Prochlorperazine is a phenothiazine derivative indicated for the control of severe nausea and vomiting. Calming these symptoms may also reduce some of the pain and anxiety the patient is experiencing.[1]

4. **B. Analysis.** Vomiting results in depletion of both fluid reserve and electrolytes. Serial vital signs, as well as orthostatic blood pressure and pulse measurement, are indicated in the monitoring of this patient, as is an accurate record of intake and output.

5. **D. Evaluation.** When intake is nearly equivalent to output, urine specific gravity is normal, and electrolyte balance is maintained, the parameters for adequate fluid volume have been satisfied.

6. **A. Assessment.** Abdominal examination of the patient with appendicitis reveals point tenderness over the right lower quadrant with rebound because of peritoneal irritation. When the acute process has been present for some time, ileus may develop, causing bowel sounds to be diminished or absent. In general, however, bowel sounds are of little help in establishing the diagnosis.[5]

7. **C. Analysis.** Appendicitis is an inflammation and/or obstruction of the vermiform appendix, a blind pouch extending from the proximal part of the cecum. This condition can lead to ischemia of the appendix, resulting in necrosis, perforation, and subsequent peritonitis or abscess formation. In one study, the appendix had already perforated at the time of surgery in 55% of patients under 6 years of age after only 2 days of symptoms.[5]

8. **D. Intervention.** Although a 5-year-old boy is beginning to venture out into the world as he goes off to preschool, in times of crisis he still has a strong need of his parent for support. Approaching the child in a calm, quiet manner and explaining procedures in understandable terms will allay the fears of both parent and child.

9. **A. Assessment.** The first response here would be to recheck the patient, alert for a decreased blood pressure, an increased pulse, or a rising temperature. An increase in the respiratory rate may be significant as peritoneal irritation increases, but this is difficult to evaluate in a tearful child. The other interventions may be appropriate, but only after a search for evidence of a worsening condition has been conducted.

10. **B. Intervention.** Cephalosporins, like all antibiotics, are very irritating in concentrated form. They are less likely to cause venous inflammation if they are diluted and infused over a 20- to 30-minute period.

11. **C. Intervention.** Current medications assist the nurse in gaining helpful information regarding the patient's past medical history and will need to be identified. However, this patient's clinical presentation indicates that some acute process is taking place. Acute anterior myocardial infarction may mimic this appearance and must be recognized early, before life-threatening dysrhythmias ensue.

12. **D. Assessment.** Acute pancreatitis is found in conjunction with biliary tract disease in more than 50% of patients. Another well-known indicator is alcohol abuse. Although the actual etiology of the disease is not clear, whatever the cause, the primary lesion is a chemical inflammation caused by pancreatic enzymes and secretions, which leads to necrosis of gland cells.[6]

13. **A. Analysis.** The pancreas responds to the chemical inflammation initially by edema, and as much as 30% of plasma volume may be entrapped in the gland.[6] In addition, large volumes of fluid may pool retroperitoneally, thus contributing to hypovolemia.[5]

14. **B. Evaluation.** Fluid replacement must be accomplished with caution in patients who have any known or suspected cardiac disease. That this patient is taking antihypertensives is an indication that her cardiovasculature is not normal. The stress of this acute illness plus the rapid infusion of fluid may push a compensated heart failure over into overt cardiac decompensation.

15. **A. Assessment.** The enzyme amylase is released into the blood by the damaged pancreatic tissue. Another enzyme that is released in large amounts is lipase. Two major problems resulting from lipase release are fat necrosis of the pancreas and hypocalcemia.[6]

16. **C. Assessment.** Atherosclerosis is responsible for much of cerebrovascular and peripheral arterial disease, as well as most abdominal aortic aneurysms. This patient has two markers in his history: a cerebrovascular accident (CVA) and hypertension. The appearance of sudden acute abdominal or back pain in any patient older than 50 years of age points to an abdominal aortic aneurysm. Men are more commonly affected than women. The vast majority of these patients have known hypertension.

17. **B. Assessment.** The aortic wall is weakened at the area of plaque formation because of erosion. Local dilation occurs in the area of weakness. The dissection process is a tearing of the intimal layer of the vessel, with resulting blood leakage between the intimal and medial layers.[6]

18. **D. Intervention.** The definitive treatment of an expanding or ruptured aortic aneurysm is surgical. Insertion of at least two large-bore IV needles and a Foley catheter, as well as performance of an ECG and laboratory sample collection, must be done quickly in order to get the patient into surgery as soon as possible.

19. **D. Analysis.** Since the patient is symptomatic, it may be concluded that his aneurysm is expanding. Rupture is imminent. There may already be leakage that is tamponaded by retroperitoneal tissues.

20. **A. Evaluation.** If the patient is stable when first seen, as in this case, IV fluids should be given at a rate adequate to maintain urine output but not to elevate the patient's blood pressure. Patients who are unstable initially or who become unstable in the emergency department should be resuscitated with fluids up to a systolic pressure of 90 to 100 mm Hg.[5]

21. **B. Assessment.** Sudden onset of painless hematemesis is the hallmark sign of bleeding esophageal varices. The patient at risk for this condition is the chronic alcoholic patient with cirrhosis. Hypertension is not commonly part of the syndrome.

22. **D. Assessment.** Most esophageal varices result from progressive liver disease; fibrotic liver changes and hepatic vein obstruction result in portal hypertension, which eventually causes development of collateral circulation in adjoining organs, specifically the distal esophagus. As pressure in the portal vein rises, these collateral vessels bulge and are susceptible to rupture, causing extensive bleeding.[6]

23. **A. Analysis.** This patient's airway is of concern because he is a lethargic, intoxicated individual who is vomiting. He is at risk for aspiration and requires careful nursing measures to prevent this.

24. **C. Intervention.** In addition to providing a means for gastric suction and lavage if indicated, the Blakemore tube is equipped with esophageal and gastric balloons to tamponade bleeding at the distal esophageal sites.

25. **D. Intervention.** Because of the significant possibility of trauma to fragile varices in the lower esophagus, any adjustment in tube placement is a physician responsibility.

26. **A. Evaluation.** Although the exact mechanism of action is not understood, vitamin K is known to promote the hepatic synthesis of active prothrombin. In the patient with compromised liver function, bleeding disorders are not uncommon. A minimum of 1 to 2 hours is needed to see a response to parenteral vitamin K.[7]

27. **C. Intervention.** All of the interventions listed are important in the early care of this patient. Airway management, however, is always first.

28. **B. Assessment.** Chest and/or abdominal trauma should be considered immediately in any patient who has a history of being beaten. No audible blood pressure and significant tachycardia point to the very real possibility of occult bleeding. These vital signs are inconsistent with both head injury and cocaine toxicity.

29. **A. Assessment.** The stated respiratory rate of 48 with poor ventilatory effort is the observation that leads to this diagnosis.[8]

30. **D. Intervention.** The only absolute contraindication to peritoneal lavage is the presence of a distended bladder. Therefore a Foley catheter is inserted prior to this procedure.

31. **B. Evaluation.** A bloody lavage is 98% accurate in indicating intraabdominal bleeding and dictates surgery without delay.[2]

REFERENCES

1. Sheehy SB, Marvin JA, Jimmerson CL: *Manual of clinical trauma care: the first hour*, St Louis, 1989, Mosby–Year Book.
2. Sheehy SB: *Mosby's manual of emergency care*, ed 3, St Louis, 1990, Mosby–Year Book.
3. Mowad L, Ruhle D: *Handbook of emergency nursing: the nursing process approach*, East Norwalk, Conn, 1988, Appleton & Lange.
4. Rea R et al: *Emergency nursing core curriculum*, ed 3, Philadelphia, 1987, WB Saunders.
5. Tintinalli J: *Emergency medicine*, New York, 1988, McGraw-Hill.
6. Groer M, Shekleton M: *Basic pathophysiology*, St Louis, 1983, Mosby–Year Book.
7. Karch A, Boyd E: *Handbook of drugs*, Philadelphia, 1989, JB Lippincott.
8. Kim MJ, McFarland GK, McLane AM: *Pocket guide to nursing diagnoses*, ed 4, St Louis, 1990, Mosby–Year Book.

Chapter 2

Cardiovascular Emergencies

REVIEW OUTLINE

I. Anatomy
    A. Heart
        1. Right ventricle
        2. Left ventricle
        3. Right atrium
        4. Left atrium
        5. Valves
        6. Cardiac muscle
    B. Cardiac vasculature
        1. Superior vena cava
        2. Aortic arch
        3. Coronary arteries
        4. Inferior vena cava
        5. Pulmonary arteries
        6. Pulmonary veins

II. Physiology
    A. Preload
    B. Afterload
    C. Starling's law

III. Electrical conduction
    A. Cardiac cells
    B. Sinoatrial (SA) node
    C. Atrioventricular (AV) node
    D. Bundle of His
    E. Right bundle
    F. Left bundle
    G. Purkinje fiber

H. P wave
I.   Q wave
J.   R wave
K. ST segment
L.   T wave
IV.   Cardiovascular assessment
   A. History
      1. Chest pain differentiation
         a. Provocation and palliation
         b. Quality and intensity
         c. Region and radiation
         d. Severity
         e. Temporal: When did it start? How long has the pain been there? Is there any time it is not there?
      2. Past medical history
      3. Risk factors for cardiac disease
         a. Hypertension
         b. Pulmonary disease
         c. Previous cardiac disease
         d. Smoking
         e. Family history
         f. Diabetes
         g. Renal disease
         h. Obesity
         i.   Postmenopausal women
         j.   Personality traits
         k. Elevated blood lipids
         l.   Lack of exercise
      4. Associated signs and symptoms
         a. Syncope
         b. Weakness
         c. Nausea and vomiting
         d. Dizziness
         e. Orthopnea
         f. Dependent edema
         g. Fatigue
         h. Paroxysmal nocturnal dyspnea
      5. Identification of possible contraindications to thrombolytic therapy
         a. History of recent major surgery
         b. History of cerebral vascular disease or event

    c. Intracranial neoplasm

    d. Recent trauma

    e. Recent gastrointestinal or genitourinary bleeding

    f. Puncture of a noncompressible vessel such as the insertion of a central catheter

    g. Uncontrolled hypertension

    h. Pregnancy

    i. Menstruation

    j. Known bleeding diathesis

    k. Acute pericarditis

B. Physical examination

  1. Obvious signs and symptoms of trauma

    a. Penetrating trauma: gunshot wound, knife wound, penetrating objects

    b. Blunt trauma: bruising and abrasions of the chest wall— anterior and posterior

    c. Obvious deformity

    d. Paradoxical movement

    e. Respiratory distress

  2. Level of consciousness

  3. Patient's skin color and temperature

    a. Pallor

    b. Cyanosis

    c. Diaphoresis

  4. Jugular vein distention

  5. Hepatomegaly

  6. Rate and rhythm of respirations

  7. Palpation of peripheral pulses

  8. Auscultation of breath sounds

    a. Comparison from side to side

    b. Presence or absence of breath sounds

    c. Rales

    d. Rhonchi

    e. Wheezes

    f. Pleural friction rub

  9. Auscultation of heart sounds

    a. S_1

    b. S_2

    c. S_3

    d. S_4

e. Friction rub

f. Murmurs

g. Bruits

10. Assessment of presence of edema

a. Location

b. Pitting or nonpitting

11. Dysrhythmia recognition

12. Blood pressure evaluation

a. Hypotension

b. Hypertension

c. Variances in pulse pressure

d. Pulsus alterans

e. Comparison of blood pressure from side to side

C. Diagnostic studies or procedures

1. Electrocardiogram (ECG)

2. Chest x-ray studies

3. Serum enzyme studies

4. Cardiac catheterization

5. Pericardiocentesis

6. Needle thoracostomy

7. Chest tube insertion

8. Open thoracotomy

9. Doppler studies

10. Arteriogram

V. Related nursing diagnoses

A. Activity intolerance

B. Airway clearance, ineffective

C. Breathing pattern, ineffective

D. Cardiac output, decreased

E. Fatigue

F. Fear

G. Fluid volume deficit

H. Fluid volume excess

I. Gas exchange, impaired

J. Grieving, anticipatory

K. Injury, potential for

L. Knowledge deficit

M. Pain

N. Spiritual distress (distress of the human spirit)

O. Tissue perfusion, altered

P. Trauma, potential for

VI. Collaborative care of the patient with a cardiovascular emergency
   A. ABCDE (airway, breathing, circulation, deficit [neurological], exposure)
      1. BCLS (basic cardiac life support)
      2. ACLS (advanced cardiac life support)
      3. PALS (pediatric advanced life support)
      4. BTLS (basic trauma life support)
      5. ATLS (advanced trauma life support)
   B. Oxygen therapy
   C. Cardiac monitoring
   D. Pulse oximetry
   E. External pacemaker
   F. Transvenous pacemaker
   G. Chest tube insertion
   H. Open thoracotomy
   I. Drug therapy
      1. Vasoactive drugs
      2. Antidysrhythmics
      3. Antibiotics
      4. Analgesics
      5. Inotropic agents
      6. Thrombolytic therapy
      7. Digitalis antibodies
      8. Antihypertensive agents
      9. Calcium channel blockers
     10. Anticoagulants
   J. Defibrillation and cardioversion
   K. Pericardiocentesis
   L. Frequent assessment
   M. Arterial line insertion
   N. Swan-Ganz catheters
   O. Intraaortic balloon pump
   P. Cardiopulmonary bypass
   Q. Doppler assessment
   R. Automatic implantable cardioverter defibrillator (AICD)

VII. Specific cardiovascular emergencies
   A. Congestive heart failure, acute pulmonary edema
   B. Dysrhythmia
      1. Ventricular fibrillation

  2. Ventricular tachycardia
  3. Asystole
  4. Heart block
  5. Premature ventricular contractions (PVCs)
  6. Supraventricular tachycardia
 C. Malignant hypertension
 D. Digitalis intoxication
 E. Venous thrombosis
 F. Arterial occlusion
 G. Myocardial infarction
 H. Angina
 I. Aortic aneurysm
 J. Cardiac trauma
  1. Penetrating
   a. Gunshot wounds
   b. Stab wounds
  2. Blunt
   a. Myocardial contusion
   b. Pericardial tamponade

INTRODUCTION

*I*t has been found that diseases of the heart and the vascular system account for more deaths in the United States than any of the other causes of death combined.[1] A majority of these patients seek treatment in the emergency department. In addition, the care of these patients is continuously changing. Research has demonstrated that patients suffering from such a cardiovascular emergency as an acute myocardial infarction need to be treated as a trauma patient is treated. In other words, time and skill are of the essence in preventing additional injury to the patient's myocardium.[2,3]

Cardiovascular emergencies can have either a medical or a traumatic origin. Occasionally a patient may sustain a cardiovascular emergency of both a medical and a traumatic nature, such as in the case of the elderly patient who has an acute myocardial event that precipitates a motor vehicle crash.

The care of the patient who is experiencing a cardiovascular emergency begins with the assessment and stabilization of the patient's airway, breathing, and circulation (ABCs). The emergency nurse needs to have knowledge about the anatomy and physiology of the cardiovascular system, and these topics are included in the Review Outline at the beginning of the chapter. Advanced cardiac life support (ACLS) and pediatric advanced life support (PALS) offer guidelines for the care of both the adult and the pediatric patient who is experiencing a cardiovascular emergency.

Since the cardiovascular system affects all other body systems, inspection of the patient who is suffering from a cardiovascular emergency will encompass airway patency, breathing patterns, and perfusion. Palpation should include evaluation of both the central and the peripheral pulses. Auscultation of heart sounds, cardiac rhythm, and breath sounds should be included.

Identifying the origins of the patient's chest pain, or chest pain differentiation, presents a demanding challenge to the assessment skills of the emergency department nurse. One method that can be used to differentiate a patient's chest pain is based on four different factors: the patient's description of the pain (crushing, burning, tearing, sudden onset, location); factors that relieve the pain (stopping activity, sitting up, analgesics, relief with nitroglycerin, no relief); associated symptoms (friction rub, shortness of breath, nausea, vomiting, diaphoresis); and ECG findings (no changes, elevated ST segments, transient ST and T wave changes).[4]

Diagnostic data related to cardiovascular emergencies include an ECG, chest x-ray film, serum cardiac enzyme levels, electrolytes (particularly potassium and calcium), and Doppler studies.

Specific collaborative procedures for the patient who is suffering from a cardiovascular emergency include the insertion of chest tubes,[5] pericardiocentesis, open thoracotomy, portable extracorporeal circulation,[6] and thrombolytic therapy.[7-10] The emergency nurse needs to review the indications for each of these procedures, the nurse's role in each of these procedures, and the nursing interventions required to provide emergency nursing care to patients who are undergoing these procedures.

The care of the patient who is suffering from a cardiovascular emergency begins with an understanding of the anatomy and physiology of the cardiovascular system. The emergency nurse needs to be able to differentiate the sources of chest pain. Recognition and treatment of potentially lethal dysrhythmia is a very important component of the care provided to the patient with a cardiovascular emergency. Finally, having current knowledge about the care of the patient with acute myocardial infarction — particularly thrombolytic therapy — and recognizing and providing treatment for the patient who may have experienced blunt or penetrating cardiac trauma contribute to the emergency nurse's providing optimal care to the patient who is suffering from a cardiovascular emergency.

REVIEW QUESTIONS
Myocardial Infarction

A 53-year-old man comes to the emergency department complaining of midsternal chest pain. He is awake, alert, pale, and diaphoretic. His vital signs are blood pressure, 110/70; pulse, 88 and irregular; respiratory rate, 22; and temperature, 98.6° F.

1. The pain pattern of myocardial infarction frequently is described as:
   0   A. Tearing, radiating to the back
   0   B. Sudden, sharp, increasing with a change in position
   0   C. Sudden, crushing, radiating to the jaw and neck
   0   D. Sudden, sharp over the lung fields, increasing with inspiration

2. Thrombolytic therapy is being considered to treat this patient. All of the following would contribute to making a decision *except:*
   0   A. Serum cardiac enzyme levels
   0   B. A 12-lead ECG
   0   C. A history of cardiovascular disease
   0   D. The length of time since pain onset

3. ST elevation on a 12-lead ECG indicates:
   0   A. Infarction
   0   B. Ischemia
   0   C. Dysrhythmia
   0   D. Injury

4. The emergency nurse obtains a 12-lead ECG. There is ST elevation greater than 2 cm in leads II, III, and aV$_F$. The patient is having an acute:
   0   A. Anterior wall infarction
   0   B. Inferior wall infarction
   0   C. Posterior wall infarction
   0   D. Lateral wall infarction

5. Tissue plasminogen activator (t-PA) is ordered for this patient. In preparation for administration of thrombolytic therapy, the emergency nurse may:
   0   A. Place an external pacemaker on the patient
   0   B. Use the IV site to draw blood from
   0   C. Administer platelets to the patient
   0   D. Start a dopamine drip

6. The patient is to be transported to the cardiac catheterization unit. In preparation for transport, the emergency nurse should:
   - 0 A. Change all the patient's IV fluids to normal saline
   - 0 B. Place blood tubing on one of the IV lines
   - 0 C. Bring along a defibrillator and ACLS drugs
   - 0 D. Place a pulse oximeter on the patient

7. After the t-PA has been infused, the emergency nurse should:
   - 0 A. Purge the IV tubing to get all of the drug
   - 0 B. Draw a CBC
   - 0 C. Insert a Foley catheter
   - 0 D. Draw a PT and a PTT

8. An infusion of t-PA is administered to this patient. A common dysrhythmia associated with reperfusion is:
   - 0 A. Ventricular fibrillation
   - 0 B. Complete heart block
   - 0 C. Accelerated idioventricular rhythm
   - 0 D. Asystole

9. The most common complication of thrombolytic therapy is:
   - 0 A. Reperfusion dysrhythmia
   - 0 B. Bleeding
   - 0 C. Thrombosis
   - 0 D. Hypocalcemia

10. Because of the possibility of an intracerebral bleed occurring as the result of t-PA administration, the emergency nurse should evaluate the patient for:
   - 0 A. The presence of petechiae
   - 0 B. Changes in level of consciousness, as well as nausea and vomiting
   - 0 C. Blood in his urine
   - 0 D. Fever and chills

11. The most appropriate nursing diagnosis for the patient receiving thrombolytic therapy is:
   - 0 A. Airway clearance, ineffective
   - 0 B. Fluid volume deficit
   - 0 C. Injury, potential for
   - 0 D. Gas exchange, impaired

12. T-PA:
    0   A. Is clot specific
    0   B. Causes a lytic state
    0   C. Is not clot specific
    0   D. Has a prolonged effect on the coagulation system

A 43-year-old man comes to the emergency department complaining of chest pain for the past 12 hours. He states that it is crushing and goes down his left arm.

13. Control of chest pain is important in the patient having a myocardial infarction because:
    0   A. It may interfere with the patient's level of consciousness
    0   B. It will increase the patient's anxiety and fear
    0   C. Pain releases catecholamines and may increase myocardial damage
    0   D. Pain may cause nausea and vomiting

14. The patient states, "I do not know what this heart attack is going to do to my life." The most appropriate nursing diagnosis on which the emergency nurse should base care is:
    0   A. Fear related to the implications of the patient's illness
    0   B. Body image disturbance related to the acute myocardial infarction
    0   C. Thought processes, altered, related to chest pain
    0   D. Spiritual distress (distress of the human spirit) related to pain

15. After providing the patient with information about his condition, the emergency nurse should use which of the following to evaluate the effectiveness of the intervention?
    0   A. The patient's pulse and blood pressure increases
    0   B. The patient is able to talk about his fears
    0   C. The patient states that he wants to be alone
    0   D. The patient says that he does not want to see his family

A 60-year-old patient is diagnosed as having an acute inferior wall myocardial infarction and a right ventricular infarction. He is awake and alert. The patient develops profound hypotension while in the emergency department. His vital signs are blood pressure, 80/50; pulse, 60; and respiratory rate, 32.

16. The initial management of this patient should include:
    0   A. Administration of furosemide (Lasix)
    0   B. Administration of IV fluids

0   C. Insertion of a transvenous pacemaker
0   D. Endotracheal intubation

17. A right ventricular infarct is diagnosed by:
0   A. A chest x-ray film
0   B. Placement of right-sided precordial leads
0   C. Serum cardiac enzymes
0   D. Cardiac arrest

18. Diagnosis of an acute myocardial infarction in the emergency department is based on which of the following clinical criteria?
0   A. Cardiac catheterization
0   B. Elevation of an ST segment greater than 2 cm in one lead
0   C. The patient's history and a 12-lead ECG
0   D. Pathological Q waves in two leads on the ECG

Advanced Cardiac Life Support

The rescue squad brings in a 35-year-old woman found lying on the sidewalk. The patient is receiving full CPR.

19. When the patient is placed on the monitor, the following rhythm is found. What is it?

V_1

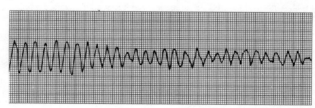

0   A. Sinus rhythm
0   B. Ventricular tachycardia
0   C. Ventricular fibrillation
0   D. Asystole

20. The patient has been defibrillated twice and remains in the same rhythm. What should the emergency team do next?
0   A. Check a pulse and defibrillate at 360 watts/sec
0   B. Continue CPR until an IV line is established

0   C. Intubate and hyperventilate the patient

0   D. Give the patient 10 mg of epinephrine

21. The patient's monitor shows a rhythm, but a pulse cannot be palpated. What interventions should the emergency nurse consider?

0   A. Stopping CPR

0   B. Giving two ampules of sodium bicarbonate

0   C. Giving calcium chloride

0   D. Giving the patient a fluid bolus

• • •

22. A 52-year-old man comes to the emergency department complaining of chest pain. When placed on the monitor, he is found to be in an irregular rhythm. What rhythm is he in?

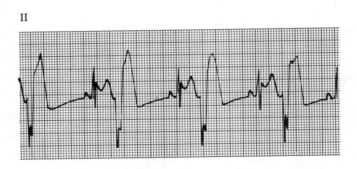

II

0   A. Ventricular tachycardia

0   B. Ventricular bigeminy

0   C. Asystole

0   D. Complete heart block

23. This patient's rhythm is treated with:

0   A. Atropine, 0.5 mg IV push

0   B. Lidocaine, 1 mg/kg IV push

0   C. Sodium bicarbonate, 1 mEq/kg IV push

0   D. An external pacemaker

24. An 80-year-old man is brought to the emergency department after having collapsed while mowing the lawn. When his family found him, he was

apneic and pulseless, and CPR was initiated. When the patient arrives in the emergency department, the monitor shows the following rhythm:

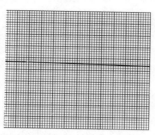

- 0   A. Asystole
- 0   B. Ventricular tachycardia
- 0   C. Sinus rhythm
- 0   D. Electrical mechanical dissociation

25. The patient is intubated, but an IV line has not yet been established. All of the following drugs can be placed down the endotracheal tube *except:*
- 0   A. Lidocaine
- 0   B. Atropine
- 0   C. Naloxone
- 0   D. Sodium bicarbonate

26. A 60-year-old woman is brought to the emergency department after having passed out at home. When the patient is placed on the monitor, the following rhythm is found:

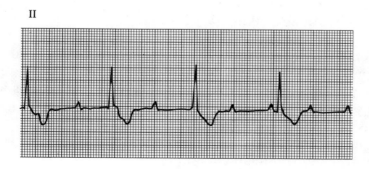

- 0   A. Asystole
- 0   B. First-degree heart block

0   C. Third-degree heart block
0   D. Sinus rhythm

27. A common complication of external pacing in the awake patient is:
    0   A. Failure to capture through the patient's skin
    0   B. Failure of pacing pads to stick to the patient's chest wall
    0   C. Pain from muscle spasms induced by the pacemaker
    0   D. Shortness of breath because the patient has to lie flat during
        pacing

28. An 18-year-old woman comes to the emergency department complain-
    ing of a "funny" feeling in her chest and shortness of breath. The
    patient's blood pressure is 80/60; her pulse is 200. Valsalva maneuvers
    do not decrease or change the patient's rhythm. Which of the following
    drugs may be ordered to treat this dysrhythmia?

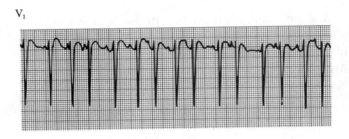

    0   A. Epinephrine, 1 mg/kg IV push
    0   B. Atropine, 1 mg IV push
    0   C. Adenosine, 6 mg IV push
    0   D. Procainamide, 50 mg IV push

29. A 6-month-old infant is brought to the emergency department because
    of respiratory distress. The baby's pulse is over 230 beats per minute.
    The mother states that the child has not been ill and that this incident
    started suddenly. The baby is awake, restless, and cyanotic. The physi-
    cian has decided to cardiovert the baby.
        The emergency nurse would calculate the watt-seconds to be used to
    cardiovert the baby using the following:
    0   A. 2 J/kg
    0   B. 0.5 J/kg
    0   C. 3 J/kg
    0   D. 0.25 J/kg

30. Because of possible cardiovascular collapse, which of the following drugs should not be given to infants who are in a supraventricular rhythm?
0   A. Epinephrine
0   B. Atropine
0   C. Verapamil
0   D. Lidocaine

31. For the patient who has an implanted cardioverter defibrillator in place and who needs to be defibrillated, how should the paddles be placed?
0   A. The patient should not be defibrillated
0   B. The paddles should be placed on the apex and sternum
0   C. The paddles should be placed anteriorly and posteriorly
0   D. The patient's chest should be opened for internal defibrillation

Hypertension

A 37-year-old black man is brought to the emergency department by his family. He is complaining of a headache and blurred vision. He has no known medical problems and is not taking any medication. His vital signs are blood pressure, 220/134; pulse, 100; and respiratory rate, 22.

32. A hypertensive crisis is occurring when the patient's diastolic blood pressure is greater than:
0   A. 90 mm Hg
0   B. 100 mm Hg
0   C. 120 mm Hg
0   D. 130 mm Hg

33. Signs and symptoms of complications related to hypertension include:
0   A. A diastolic blood pressure of 80 mm Hg
0   B. Right ventricular hypertrophy
0   C. Impaired renal function
0   D. Normal potassium levels

34. The emergency physician orders labetalol, 20 mg IV push, for the patient. A possible side effect of this drug is:
0   A. Orthostatic hypotension
0   B. Tachycardia
0   C. Excessive salivation
0   D. Headache

•   •   •

35. A patient with newly diagnosed hypertension is prescribed hydrochlorothiazide (Hydrodiuril), 50 mg b.i.d., by the emergency physician. The patient states, "I have never taken any medicine for my blood pressure before." The emergency nurse should base discharge instructions on which of the following nursing diagnoses?

   0   A. Knowledge deficit related to the use of a new drug for a newly diagnosed disease process
   0   B. Body image disturbance related to physical changes that occur with hypertension
   0   C. Thought processes, altered, related to the cerebral changes brought about by chronic hypertension
   0   D. Family processes, altered, related to the need for a family member to take a new medication

36. The emergency nurse provides information to the patient about his disease process and refers him for follow-up care. Which of the following measures could the emergency nurse use to evaluate the effectiveness of this intervention?

   0   A. The patient returns to the emergency department for follow-up care
   0   B. The patient keeps his appointment at the hypertension clinic
   0   C. The patient does not take his medicine and returns in a hypertensive crisis
   0   D. The patient leaves his referral information at the emergency department

Congestive Heart Failure

An 82-year-old woman is brought to the emergency department by the rescue squad. She was woken from her sleep by severe shortness of breath and chest pain. On arrival in the emergency department, she is awake, short of breath, diaphoretic, and pale. Her vital signs are blood pressure, 160/100; pulse, 120; and respiratory rate, 32. Rales are auscultated in both lung fields.

37. Which of the following disease processes most often contributes to congestive heart failure in the adult patient?

   0   A. Cardiomyopathy
   0   B. Congenital cardiac disease
   0   C. Mitral valve prolapse
   0   D. Hypertension

38. The emergency physician orders 1 inch of nitropaste to be applied to the patient's chest. Vasodilators are useful in congestive heart failure because they:

   0 A. Increase preload and afterload
   0 B. Cause diuresis
   0 C. Decrease preload
   0 D. Increase afterload

39. Morphine, 2 mg, is administered by IV push by the emergency nurse. Morphine is an effective drug for the patient with congestive heart failure because it:

   0 A. Produces respiratory arrest
   0 B. Produces myocardial depression
   0 C. Increases the patient's heart rate
   0 D. Reduces venous return

40. The patient is given 40 mg of furosemide (Lasix) for diuresis. One intervention the emergency nurse could perform to decrease patient exertion would be to:

   0 A. Insert a Foley catheter
   0 B. Place the patient in Trendelenburg position
   0 C. Give the patient oxygen by nasal cannula
   0 D. Place a pulse oximeter on the patient

41. The patient's blood gas results are as follows: pH, 7.37; Pco_2, 25; Po_2, 60; and HCO_3, 18. Using the data collected from these blood gas results, which of the following nursing diagnoses would the emergency nurse use to base care on?

   0 A. Fluid volume deficit related to diuresis with furosemide
   0 B. Gas exchange, impaired, related to the patient's congestive heart failure
   0 C. Activity intolerance related to the low Po_2
   0 D. Tissue integrity, impaired, related to the patient's acute congestive heart failure

42. The patient's oxygen source is changed to a 100% nonrebreather mask. In addition to arterial blood gases (ABGs), what other data could the emergency nurse use to elevate the patient's condition?

   0 A. Level of consciousness
   0 B. Hemoglobin and hematocrit

    0   C. Urinary output
    0   D. Palpation of peripheral pulses

Thrombophlebitis and Arteriovascular Disease

A 25-year-old woman comes to the emergency department complaining of pain and swelling in her right calf.

43. Risk factors that would contribute to the development of thrombophlebitis in this patient include all of the following *except:*
    0   A. Wearing antiembolic stockings
    0   B. Taking oral contraceptives
    0   C. Sepsis
    0   D. Prolonged bed rest

44. Signs and symptoms of venous thrombosis include:
    0   A. Nonpalpable peripheral pulses
    0   B. Lack of pain in the affected extremity
    0   C. Absence of Homans' sign
    0   D. An extremity that is red, hot, and swollen

An 88-year-old man is brought to the emergency department because of severe pain in his left leg.

45. The physical examination of a patient with an acute arterial occlusion would reveal:
    0   A. Palpable peripheral pulses
    0   B. A red, warm extremity
    0   C. A pale, cold extremity
    0   D. Presence of Homans' sign

46. The emergency nurse should prepare the patient with an acute arterial occlusion for:
    0   A. Surgery
    0   B. Anticoagulant therapy with coumadin
    0   C. Application of ice to, and elevation of, the affected extremity
    0   D. Application of antiembolic hose

47. The appropriate nursing diagnosis on which the emergency nurse should base the care of this patient is:
    0   A. Gas exchange, impaired, related to an acute arterial occlusion

0 B. Tissue perfusion, altered (peripheral), related to an acute arterial occlusion

0 C. Fluid volume deficit related to an acute arterial occlusion

0 D. Disuse syndrome, potential for, related to an acute arterial occlusion of a lower extremity

Digitalis Toxicity

A 3-year-old child has ingested his grandmother's digitalis. The family is unsure about the amount of pills the child has taken. He is currently awake, nauseated, and vomiting.

48. The most common dysrhythmia seen in patients with digitalis toxicity who do not have cardiac disease is:

0 A. Ventricular bigeminy

0 B. Ventricular tachycardia

0 C. Sinus bradycardia

0 D. AV junctional tachycardia

49. The child's monitor shows a sinus bradycardia. He progresses to a third-degree block with a blood pressure of 70/40. Which drug should the emergency team administer?

0 A. Lidocaine, 1 mg/kg IV push

0 B. Isoproterenol drip

0 C. Atropine, 0.4 mg IV push

0 D. Epinephrine, 0.1 mg/kg

50. Digibind is being considered to treat this child. All of the following are indications for the use of digoxin-specific antibody fragments *except:*

0 A. Cardiac arrest from digitalis toxicity

0 B. Bradyarrhythmias unresponsive to atropine

0 C. Severe hyperkalemia

0 D. Conversion to sinus rhythm after atropine

•   •   •

51. Plants that contain cardiac glycosides include all of the following *except:*

0 A. Foxglove plant

0 B. Lily of the valley

0 C. Ramp

0 D. Hellebore

Cardiac Trauma

A 24-year-old man is brought to the emergency department following an accident in which he was struck by a car while riding his bicycle. The patient was thrown from the bike, landing on his chest. He was wearing a helmet. On arrival in the emergency department, the patient is awake, moving all his extremities, and complaining of midsternal chest pain. His vital signs are blood pressure, 100/79; pulse, 132; and respiratory rate, 28.

52. The most common sign or symptom associated with myocardial contusion is:
- 0   A. Sinus tachycardia
- 0   B. Pericardial effusion
- 0   C. Chest pain referred to the shoulder
- 0   D. Hemothorax

53. The initial evaluation of the patient with a suspected myocardial contusion in the emergency department should include:
- 0   A. A MUGA scan
- 0   B. Clotting studies
- 0   C. A 12-lead ECG
- 0   D. Serial hemoglobin and hematocrit

•   •   •

54. Beck's triad includes:
- 0   A. Increased blood pressure, distended neck veins, and muffled heart sounds
- 0   B. Decreased blood pressure, distended neck veins, and muffled heart sounds
- 0   C. Decreased blood pressure, flat neck veins, and audible heart sounds
- 0   D. Increased blood pressure, flat neck veins, and muffled heart sounds

55. A 24-year-old man has been brought to the emergency department with a stab wound in his midsternum. Initially awake, he has become unresponsive. He has a palpable pulse. The emergency nurse should prepare the patient for:
- 0   A. Insertion of a trauma catheter
- 0   B. Insertion of bilateral chest tubes
- 0   C. Emergency thoracotomy
- 0   D. Insertion of a CVP line

56. A 19-year-old woman is brought to the emergency department after having been involved in a head-on collision with a truck. She was entrapped for over an hour and has obvious signs of severe chest trauma. All of the following would indicate an aortic injury *except:*

0   A. Chest wall bruising
0   B. A first rib fracture
0   C. The trachea in the midline
0   D. Paraplegia

ANSWERS

1. **C. Assessment.** The pain pattern described by the patient having a myocardial infarction is usually sudden in onset, crushing, and substernal; the pain may radiate to the patient's neck, jaw, and back.[4]

2. **A. Assessment.** Serum cardiac enzyme levels can provide information about the evolution and resolution of injury to the myocardium. The information these tests can provide, however, is generally not available in the emergency department, and waiting for it could delay important treatment, such as thrombolytic therapy.[4]

3. **D. Assessment.** ST segment elevation indicates injury; T wave inversion indicates ischemia; and pathological Q waves indicate infarction.[2]

4. **B. Assessment.** ST elevation in leads II, III, and aV_F is indicative of an inferior infarction.[11] ST elevation in V_1, V_2, and V_3 is indicative of an anterior infarction. ST elevation in leads I, aV_1, V_5, and V_6 is indicative of a lateral infarction. Leads showing wave changes in V_1 and V_2, a tall broad initial R wave, ST segment depression, and a tall upright T wave would indicate a posterior infarction.[12]

5. **B. Intervention.** Using the IV site to draw blood from will decrease the potential for additional sites that may bleed during the administration of thrombolytics.[13]

6. **C. Intervention.** Because of the potential for reperfusion dysrhythmia during the administration of thrombolytics, the emergency nurse needs to be prepared by bringing along a defibrillator and ACLS drugs.[12]

7. **A. Intervention.** To ensure that all of the medicine has been infused, it is recommended that the tubing be purged after the infusion.[8]

8. **C. Evaluation.** Accelerated idioventricular rhythm is frequently associated with reperfusion. The usual rate is 60 to 100 beats per minute.[9]

9. **B. Assessment.** The most common complication of thrombolytic therapy is bleeding. Intracranial hemorrhage is the most dangerous complication of thrombolytic therapy.[10]

10. **B. Evaluation.** Since intracranial hemorrhage is one of the most serious

complications of thrombolytic therapy, it is important that the emergency nurse assess the patient for changes in level of consciousness, nausea and vomiting, headache, and confusion.[9]

11. **C. Analysis.** Because the patient is receiving a drug that has several serious potential side effects, the emergency nurse's care needs to be directed at preventing any injury that could result. Examples of this are drawing blood from the IV site, minimizing the number of IV sites, minimizing the number of punctures, and performing invasive procedures such as Foley catheter insertion before the administration of the drug.[9]

12. **A. Assessment.** T-PA is clot specific. It is a direct activator of plasminogen. Urokinase and streptokinase cause lytic states.[7]

13. **C. Intervention.** Pain stimulates the release of catecholamines, which can lead to additional oxygen demands on an already compromised myocardium.[14]

14. **A. Analysis.** The defining characteristics of this nursing diagnosis include increased tension, verbalization of fear, decreased self-assurance, and sympathetic stimulation. A related factor that would contribute to the use of this nursing diagnosis on which to base emergency nursing care is the fact that the patient is separated from his support system in a potentially life-threatening situation.[15]

15. **B. Evaluation.** One of the expected outcomes for emergency nursing interventions related to this diagnosis would be that the patient would be able to verbalize his feelings about the source of his fear and about what he is able to do to deal with it.[14]

16. **B. Intervention.** Right ventricular infarction occurs in about 40% of patients who suffer an inferior wall myocardial infarction. Treatment for the hypotension that occurs with right ventricular infarction is the administration of fluids.[2]

17. **B. Assessment.** Right ventricular infarcts are diagnosed by the placement of right-sided precordial leads.[2]

18. **C. Assessment.** The diagnosis of an acute myocardial infarction is based on three factors: history, clinical examination, and a 12-lead ECG. The history and clinical evaluation help the emergency nurse identify risk factors for heart disease, such as smoking and hypertension. A 12-lead ECG may show ischemia, injury, or infarction. Enzyme analysis (not generally available in the emergency department) will show the extent of damage that has occurred.[2]

19. **C. Assessment.** Ventricular fibrillation.

20. **A. Intervention.** The emergency team should check a pulse and then defibrillate the patient with 360 watts/sec. The ACLS algorithm for ven-

tricular fibrillation is as follows: defibrillate the patient with 200 watts/sec and check a pulse; if no pulse is palpated, defibrillate with 200 to 300 watts/sec and check a pulse; if no pulse is palpated, defibrillate at 360 watts/sec and then continue CPR if no pulse is palpated.[16]

21. **D. Intervention.** When electrical activity is detected but no pulse is palpated, the patient is in electromechanical dissociation (EMD). When the patient is in EMD, the emergency nurse needs to consider the possibility of hypovolemia, cardiac tamponade, tension pneumothorax, acidosis, pulmonary embolism, and hypoxemia, as well as what interventions could be used to correct any of these possible origins of EMD.[15]

22. **B. Assessment.** Ventricular bigeminy.

23. **B. Intervention.** The patient would be treated with lidocaine, 1 mg/kg.[15]

24. **A. Assessment.** Asystole.

25. **D. Intervention.** Lidocaine, atropine, naloxone, and epinephrine can be put down the endotracheal tube. Valium, while not a cardiac drug, can also be given down the endotracheal tube.[15]

26. **C. Assessment.** Third-degree heart block.

27. **C. Evaluation.** A common problem with the use of an external pacemaker in the awake patient is pain from the muscle spasms that occur from the pacemaker. Patients may need to be sedated until a transvenous pacemaker can be placed.[15]

28. **C. Intervention.** Adenosine slows conduction time through the AV node. It is indicated for the treatment of paroxysmal supraventricular tachycardia because it can interrupt the reentry pathway and restore sinus rhythm.[17]

29. **B. Intervention.** Synchronized cardioversion is the treatment of choice for a child with unstable tachydysrhythmia. The recommended dose is 0.5 to 1 J/kg.[18]

30. **C. Intervention.** Cardiovascular collapse has been reported in infants when verapamil has been used.[17]

31. **C. Intervention.** The paddle position for the patient who has an implanted cardioverter defibrillator is the anterior/posterior position.[19]

32. **D. Assessment.** A hypertensive crisis is defined as a diastolic blood pressure greater than 130 mm Hg. This constitutes an emergent patient problem.[20]

33. **C. Assessment.** Complications of hypertension include papilledema, left ventricular hypertrophy, congestive heart failure, impaired renal function, and intracranial or subarachnoid hemorrhage.[19]

34. **A. Evaluation.** Side effects of labetalol include orthostatic hypotension at the beginning of therapy, facial flushing, dry mouth, bradycardia, and fatigue.[21]

35. **A. Analysis.** The defining characteristics of this nursing diagnosis include verbalization of inadequate information about one's illness and the patient's requesting information about the disease process. Related factors include lack of exposure to accurate information, lack of motivation to learn, and cultural and language barriers.[14]

36. **B. Evaluation.** The expected outcome for nursing interventions related to this diagnosis would be that the patient would follow through as instructed.[14]

37. **D. Assessment.** The most common cause of congestive heart failure in the adult patient is hypertension.[22]

38. **C. Intervention.** Nitropaste is a vasodilator that decreases preload. Vasodilators, however, do not affect afterload.[21]

39. **D. Intervention.** Morphine reduces venous return by venodilation. It also reduces the respiratory rate and can decrease the patient's anxiety.[23]

40. **A. Intervention.** Inserting a Foley catheter in the patient who is being diuresed will help decrease patient exertion, as well as provide a method for the emergency nurse to keep an accurate record of output for the patient.

41. **B. Analysis.** Based on the data provided by the blood gases, the patient is hypoxic, probably as a result of impairment of gas exchange. Related factors contributing to this nursing diagnosis include alveolar capillary membrane changes and altered capacity of the blood to carry oxygen.[14]

42. **A. Evaluation.** Defining characteristics of gas exchange, impaired, include confusion, restlessness, hypoxia, and irritability. Evaluation of the patient's level of consciousness would provide information about the effect of 100% oxygen by mask.[14]

43. **A. Assessment.** Risk factors relating to the development of venous thrombosis include medications such as oral contraceptives, prolonged bed rest, trauma, varicose veins, sepsis, and stasis.[22]

44. **D. Assessment.** Signs and symptoms of venous thrombosis include swelling; a red, warm extremity; the presence of Homans' sign; and pain that may be aggravated by walking.[22]

45. **C. Assessment.** The physical examination of an extremity that has an acute arterial occlusion would show a cool, pale limb; pain; changes in motor and sensory function; lack of pulses distal to the occlusion; and slow capillary filling.[22]

46. **A. Intervention.** The treatment for acute arterial occlusion is surgical removal of the clot, or embolectomy. The quicker the occlusion is relieved, the better the patient will do. However, if surgery is delayed, the patient may be started on a regimen of heparin.[22]

47. **B. Analysis.** The defining characteristics of this nursing diagnosis in-

clude decreased or absent arterial pulses, pale extremities, cold extremities, loss of motor/sensory function, and pain.[14]

48. **C. Assessment.** Digitalis toxicity can cause numerous types of cardiac dysrhythmia. For the patient who does not have preexisting cardiac disease, such as the pediatric patient, AV block and bradyarrhythmias are common. For the patient with cardiovascular disease, tachyarrhythmias are more likely to occur.[24]

49. **C. Intervention.** Atropine is the drug of choice. The recommended dose is 10 to 30 µg/kg up to 0.4 mg.[23]

50. **D. Intervention.** Digibind, or digoxin-specific antibody fragments, is indicated for the treatment of life-threatening digitalis overdose. Complications of digitalis overdose include shock, cardiac arrest, ventricular tachycardia, ventricular fibrillation, and bradyarrhythmias refractory to atropine.[23]

51. **C. Assessment.** Plant toxicity can be a source of many types of problems. Some plants contain toxins that affect the heart in the same manner as cardiac glycosides do. These include the foxglove plant, lily of the valley, and hellebore.[25]

52. **A. Assessment.** The most common sign or symptom of myocardial contusion is sinus tachycardia. Other signs and symptoms of myocardial contusion include severe chest pain, chest wall contusion, hypotension, and dyspnea.[19,21]

53. **C. Evaluation.** The patient with chest trauma needs to have a 12-lead ECG. Enzymes may be helpful, but the information may not be available in a timely manner.[19,21]

54. **B. Assessment.** Beck's triad includes decreased blood pressure, distended jugular veins, and muffled heart sounds. These signs may be indicative of cardiac tamponade.[19]

55. **C. Intervention.** Thoracotomy is indicated for penetrating cardiac trauma, tension pneumothorax, and crush injuries to the chest.[19]

56. **C. Assessment.** Indications of aortic injury include first and second rib fractures, signs of hypovolemic shock, tracheal deviation to the right, chest wall bruising, paraplegia, and sternal fracture.[19]

REFERENCES

1. Frank I: Emergency nursing care of cardiac patients: questions and answers for the 1990s, *JEN* 16:183-184, 1990.
2. Colletti R: Diagnosis of acute myocardial infarction in the emergency department, *JEN* 16:187-190, 1990.
3. Martin JS et al: Early triage and treatment of the acute myocardial infarction patient: how fast is fast? *JEN* 16:195-202, 1990.
4. Belle-Isle C: Patient selection and administration of thrombolytic therapy, *JEN* 15:155-164, 1989.

5. Jordan K: Chest trauma, *Nursing 90* 20:34-42, 1990.

6. Brown C: Portable extracorporeal circulation: a new standard in myocardial infarction care? *JEN* 16:226-228, 1990.

7. Henderson E: Thrombolytic therapy in acute myocardial infarction: an overview, *JEN* 15:145-151, 1989.

8. Aghababian R: Role of thrombolytic therapy in emergency care, *JEN* 15:152-155, 1989.

9. Magee M: Nursing care of the patient receiving thrombolytic therapy, *JEN* 15:165-173, 1989.

10. Bennett K, Grines C: Current controversies in patient selection for thrombolytic therapy, *JEN* 16:191-194, 1990.

11. Conover MB: *Pocket guide to electrocardiography,* ed 2, St Louis, 1990, Mosby–Year Book.

12. Kitt S: Cardiac emergencies. In Kitt S, Kaiser J, editors: *Emergency nursing: a physiologic and clinical perspective,* Philadelphia, 1990, WB Saunders.

13. Ernst JK: Case review: thrombolysis in acute myocardial infarction, *JEN* 16:212-218, 1990.

14. Carlson JH et al: *Nursing diagnosis: a case study approach,* Philadelphia, 1991, WB Saunders.

15. McFarland GK and McFarlane EA: *Nursing diagnosis and intervention: planning for patient care,* St Louis, 1989, Mosby–Year Book.

16. American Heart Association: *Advanced cardiac life support,* Dallas, 1988, The Association.

17. Pharmacology literature from Lyphomed, Inc, Rosemont, Ill.

18. American Heart Association: *Pediatric advanced life support,* Dallas, 1988, The Association.

19. Schuster DM: Patients with an implanted cardioverter: a new challenge, *JEN* 16:219-225, 1990.

20. Sheehy SB: *Mosby's manual of emergency care,* ed 3, St Louis, 1990, Mosby–Year Book.

21. Karb VB, Queener SF, Freeman JB: *Handbook of drugs for nursing practice,* St Louis, 1989, Mosby–Year Book.

22. Thomas HA, O'Connor R, Hoffman G: *Emergency medicine: self-assessment and review,* ed 2, St Louis, 1988, Mosby–Year Book.

23. Cosgriff JH, Anderson DL: *The practice of emergency care,* New York, 1984, JB Lippincott.

24. Manolio TA: Digitalis. In Noji EK, Kelen GD: *Manual of toxicologic emergencies,* St Louis, 1989, Mosby–Year Book.

25. Edgerton PH: Symptoms of digitalis-like toxicity in a family after accidental ingestion of lily of the valley plant, *JEN* 15:220-223, 1989.

Chapter 3

Dental, Ear, Nose, and Throat Emergencies

REVIEW OUTLINE

I. Anatomy and physiology
    A. Anatomical structures
        1. Oral cavity and contents
        2. Deciduous and permanent teeth
        3. Pharynx
        4. Larynx
        5. Salivary glands
        6. Thyroid cartilage and gland
        7. Cricoid cartilage and membrane
        8. Trachea
        9. Mastoid process
        10. Nose, nasal cavity, and contents
        11. Four paranasal sinuses
        12. Temporomandibular joint (TMJ)
        13. External, middle, and inner ear
        14. Cranial nerves
    B. Physiology
        1. Process of taste
        2. Process of hearing
        3. Process of smell
        4. Process of mastication
        5. Process of swallowing
II. Assessment

A. Primary survey
  1. ABCDE (airway, breathing, circulation, deficit [neurological], exposure)
  2. Stabilization
B. Secondary survey
  1. History of illness or injury
     a. Mechanism and time
     b. AMPLE history
        (1) Allergies
        (2) Medications
        (3) Past medical history
        (4) Last meal
        (5) Events or treatment prior to arrival
  2. Chief complaint
     a. Pain: PQRST
        (1) Provocation
        (2) Quality
        (3) Radiation
        (4) Severity
        (5) Timing
     b. Bleeding
     c. Shortness of breath
     d. Edema, ecchymosis
     e. Foreign body
     f. Asymmetry
     g. Fever, chills
     h. Nausea, vomiting
     i. Dysphasia, dysphagia
     j. Paresthesia
     k. Foul odor and/or taste in mouth
     l. Loss of hearing
     m. Tinnitus, vertigo
     n. Trismus
     o. Loss of smell
     p. Deformity, dislocation
  3. Physical examination
     a. General appearance
     b. Teeth
        (1) Number and condition of teeth
        (2) Dental prosthesis

        (3) Gaps between existing teeth
- c. Gingiva, oral mucosa, lips, oropharynx, tongue, floor of mouth, hard and soft palates, and salivary glands
  - (1) Symmetry
  - (2) Abnormalities
- d. External ear and canal
  - (1) Position
  - (2) Blood or cerebrospinal fluid (CSF) drainage
- e. Tympanic membrane
  - (1) Intact
  - (2) Abnormalities
- f. External nose
  - (1) Position, size, symmetry
  - (2) Blood or CSF drainage
- g. Internal nose
  - (1) Septum, turbinates, mucosa
  - (2) Abnormalities
- h. Neck
  - (1) Symmetry of structures
  - (2) Abnormalities
- i. Palpation
  - (1) Symmetry
  - (2) Localized point tenderness
  - (3) Abnormal mobility
  - (4) Crepitus
  - (5) Mobility of teeth
  - (6) TMJ mobility

III. Diagnostic studies or procedures
- A. Radiology
- B. Laboratory
- C. Visualization
  1. Pharyngeal mirror
  2. Tongue blades
  3. Otoscope
  4. Nasal speculum
  5. Laryngeal mirror
  6. Suction

IV. Related nursing diagnoses
- A. Anxiety
- B. Airway clearance, ineffective

C. Fluid volume deficit (actual or potential)
D. Infection, potential for
E. Nutrition, altered
F. Pain
G. Sensory/perceptual alterations

INTRODUCTION

Dental, ear, nose, and throat emergencies are frequently not life-threatening conditions. To the patient coming to the emergency department with a chief complaint involving one of these structures, an emergent situation exists because the patient feels he or she *must* have the condition alleviated immediately. It is important for the emergency nurse to realize the patient's perception of an emergent situation and to intervene rapidly. By doing so, the nurse will meet the patient's needs and expectations, as well as sow the seeds of trust. Patients with dental, ear, nose, and throat emergencies frequently need education and referral to a specialist as part of their emergency care. They are most likely to follow recommendations when they trust the emergency personnel.

Dental, ear, nose, and throat emergencies are emergent when they have the potential to obstruct the airway, cause hypovolemia, or cause permanent sensory loss.

REVIEW QUESTIONS
Odontalgia

Mr. Brown, a 19-year-old man, comes to the emergency department at 3 AM complaining of a severe toothache (odontalgia) of 1 week's duration. His vital signs are blood pressure, 130/80; pulse, 90; and respiratory rate, 18. His skin is warm, dry, and pink.

1. The initial history should focus on the patient's:
   - 0   A. Nutrition
   - 0   B. Pain
   - 0   C. Elimination
   - 0   D. Sleep

2. The appropriate nursing diagnosis applicable to Mr. Brown is:
   - 0   A. Pain

  0 B. Fluid volume deficit
  0 C. Thought processes, altered
  0 D. Swallowing, impaired

3. The most appropriate nursing action would be to administer an:
  0 A. Antibiotic
  0 B. Antiemetic
  0 C. Analgesic
  0 D. Antiinflammatory

4. Forty-five minutes after administration, Mr. Brown tells the nurse that the pain medication is not working. The nurse knows that the onset of action of the particular medication administered should have begun by this time and suspects:
  0 A. The patient is exhibiting drug-seeking behavior
  0 B. The cause of the toothache is advanced dental caries and additional pain medication may be required
  0 C. The patient is desperate for sleep and wants to be sure he can do so when he gets home
  0 D. The wrong type of pain medication may have been ordered

Earache

A 1-year-old, Baby White, is brought to the emergency department by her parents with complaints of fever, irritability, vomiting, and diarrhea. The parents relate that Baby White has a history of frequent ear infections.

5. The classic sign of an earache in a child this age is:
  0 A. Verbal complaints of pain
  0 B. Pulling at the ear
  0 C. Chewing on cold objects
  0 D. Chewing on warm objects

6. Further assessment reveals a 1-year-old with hot, moist skin and a purulent nasal discharge. Her vital signs are pulse, 150; respiratory rate, 32; and temperature (rectal), 103.2° F. The initial nursing diagnosis for Baby White should be:
  0 A. Hyperthermia
  0 B. Anxiety
  0 C. Airway clearance, ineffective
  0 D. Swallowing, impaired

7. Baby White's medical diagnosis is acute otitis media. Initial nursing interventions should include:
   - 0   A. Administering an antipyretic
   - 0   B. Administering an antibiotic
   - 0   C. Administering an analgesic
   - 0   D. All of the above

Nosebleed (Fracture)

Ms. Lee, a 27-year-old woman with severe epistaxis, is brought to the emergency department by the rescue squad. She was the unrestrained passenger in the front seat of a car that was struck from behind. Ms. Lee reportedly struck her face on the dashboard. She is awake and oriented. Her vital signs are blood pressure, 110/70; pulse, 92; and respiratory rate, 24. She is appropriately immobilized on a backboard with a cervical collar in place. Ms. Lee has an obvious nasal deformity.

8. The initial nursing assessment should be Ms. Lee's:
   - 0   A. Airway
   - 0   B. Breathing
   - 0   C. Circulatory status
   - 0   D. Mental status

9. Ms. Lee's cervical spine is cleared; her cervical collar and backboard are removed. Her nose continues to bleed. The initial nursing intervention to stop the epistaxis should be to:
   - 0   A. Prepare for nasal packing
   - 0   B. Prepare for cauterization
   - 0   C. Apply direct pressure
   - 0   D. Provide a suction device

10. Once the bleeding stops, Ms. Lee's nose should be inspected internally for the presence of:
   - 0   A. Blood clots
   - 0   B. Bone chips
   - 0   C. A septal hematoma
   - 0   D. Purulent discharge

11. Ms. Lee requests a mirror so she can look at her nose. On observation, Ms. Lee becomes very upset. An appropriate nursing diagnosis would be:
   - 0   A. Hopelessness
   - 0   B. Coping, ineffective individual

0   C. Anxiety related to possible permanent alteration in facial
      appearance
0   D. Thought processes, altered

12. Ms. Lee is referred to an ear, nose, and throat specialist for treatment of
    her nose in 48 hours when the edema has subsided. To prevent further
    epistaxis during this 48-hour period, Ms. Lee should be instructed to:
    0   A. Sleep in an upright position
    0   B. Forcefully blow her nose to remove all clots on a routine basis
    0   C. Open her mouth when sneezing
    0   D. Avoid cold food

Sore Throat

*Mr. Blue, a 31-year-old man, comes to the triage desk with complaints of a sore
throat of 5 days' duration. Mr. Blue reports he has tried throat lozenges and aspirin
for pain, but nothing has helped. His voice is muffled. The triage nurse knows that a
great majority of sore throats do not represent a serious illness.*

13. To assist in differentiating an urgent vs. nonurgent condition, the triage
    nurse should ask Mr. Blue if he has:
    0   A. Abdominal pain
    0   B. A headache
    0   C. Difficulty swallowing
    0   D. Swollen ankles

14. Mr. Blue states he has been having increasing difficulty in swallowing. He
    is immediately taken into the emergency department for care. His vital
    signs are blood pressure, 110/70; pulse, 104; respiratory rate, 28; and tem-
    perature, 102° F. While assessing his vital signs, the nurse notes that Mr.
    Blue is drooling. The initial nursing diagnosis for Mr. Blue should be:
    0   A. Body image disturbance
    0   B. Infection, potential for
    0   C. Airway clearance, ineffective (potential)
    0   D. Violence, potential for

15. Mr. Blue is diagnosed as having a peritonsillar abscess. The initial nurs-
    ing intervention for Mr. Blue should be to:
    0   A. Elevate the head of the bed 60 to 90 degrees
    0   B. Have Mr. Blue lie flat on his side
    0   C. Have Mr. Blue lie on his stomach
    0   D. Place Mr. Blue in Trendelenburg position

16. Mr. Blue is given oxygen, antibiotics, an analgesic, and an antipyretic. The nurse realizes the importance of monitoring Mr. Blue's respiratory status and, to evaluate the effectiveness of the nursing interventions, would want to see:

   0   A. Pale, diaphoretic skin

   0   B. An increase in respiratory rate

   0   C. A decrease in blood pressure

   0   D. A decrease in pulse rate

David, a 4-year-old, is brought to the emergency department by his family with a complaint of a sore throat and fever. While observing David at the triage desk, the nurse notes that he has assumed an upright position on his mother's lap, is very quiet, and is drooling. His color is pale. The nurse suspects epiglottitis.

17. The differentiation between croup and epiglottitis can be made by eliciting the onset of symptoms. Epiglottitis has a:

   0   A. Gradual onset

   0   B. Sudden onset

18. Epiglottitis is also characterized by:

   0   A. A muffled voice

   0   B. A barky cough

   0   C. A hoarse voice

   0   D. No changes in voice

19. The nurse assesses that David should receive an urgent triage status and takes measures to immediately move him into the emergency department. To move David from the triage desk and into the emergency department, the nurse should:

   0   A. Carry him into the department

   0   B. Have his mother carry him into the department

   0   C. Have him walk into the department

   0   D. Have an orderly carry him into the department

20. David is brought into the emergency department and allowed to sit on his mother's lap. His vital signs are pulse, 100; respiratory rate, 32; and temperature, (axillary), 102° F. Regarding examination of David's pharynx, the nurse should:

   0   A. Use a tongue blade

   0   B. Have the patient open his mouth and observe the pharynx with a penlight only

0   C. Have David's mother insert the tongue blade
0   D. Not examine the pharynx

21. An appropriate nursing diagnosis would be:
    0   A. Airway clearance, ineffective
    0   B. Hypothermia
    0   C. Body image disturbance
    0   D. Hopelessness

22. Antibiotic, antipyretic, and analgesic therapies are all administered. To evaluate the effectiveness of these therapies, the nurse would expect to see an:
    0   A. Increase in drooling
    0   B. Increase in pulse and respiratory rate
    0   C. Improvement in skin color
    0   D. Increase in the use of accessory muscles for breathing

ANSWERS

1. **B. Assessment.** In the early phase of odontalgia the patient may complain of a sharp, shooting pain that occurs with a hot or cold stimulus. In the later phase the patient may describe a spontaneous intense, persistent, throbbing pain with a tooth that is extremely sensitive to touch. Tooth pain is usually more intense nocturnally.

2. **A. Analysis.** Fluid volume deficit is a potential for Mr. Brown if his tooth is sensitive to hot or cold, causing him to decrease his fluid intake. However, a review of his vital signs and skin signs demonstrates that he is not dehydrated at this time.

3. **C. Intervention.** Because it is 3 AM, the patient's most obvious need is relief of pain. After this primary need is met, associated needs can be addressed.

4. **B. Evaluation.** Irreversible tooth pain is an indication that the patient may require a root canal or tooth extraction.

5. **B. Assessment.**

6. **A. Analysis.** The initial nursing diagnosis should address the patient's priority problem. For Baby White, the initial nursing concern should be her fever, since febrile children have a high potential for seizure activity.

7. **D. Intervention.** Antipyretic administration is imperative to decrease Baby White's fever. Antibiotic therapy will usually be initiated, since acute otitis media is usually preceded by an upper respiratory tract infection or

childhood disease such as measles or scarlet fever. An analgesic would be appropriate, since acute otitis media is very painful.

8. **A. Assessment.** For any trauma patient, the initial assessment should address the airway while maintaining cervical spine immobilization. Ms. Lee's mouth should be opened and observed for the presence of blood and/or broken teeth, since foreign bodies can potentially obstruct the airway. Ms. Lee's airway should especially be inspected for blood from her obvious nasal fracture.

9. **C. Intervention.** The patient may indeed require nasal packing and/or cauterization. However, direct pressure is the first nursing intervention. Suctioning may exacerbate the bleeding.

10. **C. Assessment.** A septal hematoma is a grapelike hematoma sitting on the nasal septum. It is imperative that the hematoma be recognized and drained, or septal necrosis may occur.

11. **C. Analysis.** Patients with facial fractures are frequently anxious because of a fear of permanent facial deformities.

12. **C. Intervention.** Other measures Ms. Lee should be instructed on include the following: avoid straining (lifting, stooping); avoid further nasal trauma such as the insertion of a cotton-tipped applicator; and avoid forceful nose blowing, hot liquids, and high altitudes.

13. **C. Assessment.** Patients complaining of a sore throat should be assessed for stridor, fever, dehydration, and difficulty swallowing or talking. If any of these signs or symptoms are present, the patient should be given an urgent status, since they are indicative of serious illness.

14. **C. Analysis.** Mr. Blue is exhibiting a muffled voice, reports difficulty swallowing, is drooling, and has a fever. These are all signs and symptoms of an infectious process in the throat, which should alert the nurse to the potential for airway obstruction.

15. **A. Intervention.** This is the best position for maintaining an open airway.

16. **D. Evaluation.** A return of vital signs to within normal range is an indicator of successful treatment. All other choices are indicators for reevaluation and further interventions.

17. **B. Assessment.** The onset may occur within 4 to 12 hours.

18. **A. Assessment.** A barky cough is characteristic of croup.

19. **B. Intervention.** The main objective at this time is to keep the patient as quiet and calm as possible. If the patient does indeed have epiglottitis and starts to cry, he may obstruct his airway.

20. **D. Intervention.** For any patient with suspected epiglottitis, examination of the pharynx may precipitate airway obstruction.

21. **A. Analysis.** David's drooling is an obvious sign of his inability to handle his own secretions.
22. **C. Evaluation.** Skin color is an excellent indicator of adequate oxygenation and perfusion in children.

ADDITIONAL READINGS

Boyne PJ: Early treatment of facial trauma, *Postgrad Med* 11(5):99-111, 1985.

Cantrill SV: Facial trauma and epistaxis. In Rosen P et al, editors: *Emergency medicine: concepts and clinical practice,* ed 2, St Louis, 1988, Mosby–Year Book.

Cantrill SV: Facial trauma. In Barkin RM, Rosen P, editors: *Emergency pediatrics: a guide to ambulatory care,* ed 3, St Louis, 1990, Mosby–Year Book.

Gussack GS et al: Pediatric maxillofacial trauma: unique features in diagnosis and treatment, *Laryngoscope* 97:925-930, 1987.

Kalish MA: Airway management in maxillofacial trauma, *Emerg Med Serv* 18(6):42-44, 1989.

Kitt S, Kaiser J, editors: *Emergency nursing: a physiologic and clinical perspective,* Philadelphia, 1990, WB Saunders.

Lower J: Maxillofacial trauma, *Nurs Clin North Am* 21(4):611-628, 1986.

Manson PN, Kelly KJ: Evaluation and management of the patient with facial trauma, *Emerg Med Serv* 18(6):22-30, 1989.

Rea R et al: *Emergency nursing core curriculum,* ed 3, Philadelphia, 1987, WB Saunders.

Chapter 4 _____

Environmental Emergencies

REVIEW OUTLINE

I. General management of the patient who has been affected by an environmental emergency
  A. Assess the safety of the environment
    1. Safety of the rescue crew
    2. Safety of the health care providers
    3. Control of the environment (e.g., animal, snake loose in the area)
    4. Additional hazards that may be in the environment
    5. Contact and use of appropriate authorities and experts (e.g., zoo, Environmental Protection Agency)
    6. Preparation of the emergency department for the victim(s)
  B. General patient management
    1. ABCDE (airway, breathing, circulation, deficit [neurological], exposure): exposure of the patient could be particularly important to identify the cause of the problem and any additional injuries
    2. Vital signs: blood pressure, pulse, respiratory rate, temperature
    3. History of what occurred, description of environmental surroundings, what has been done at the scene, patients at risk (e.g., alcoholic patients, homeless, young, old)
    4. Initial interventions
      a. Based on specific illness or injury
      b. Intravenous access
      c. Medications as indicated
      d. Baseline neurological assessment
      e. Consultation of appropriate authorities
      f. Wound care
II. Related nursing diagnoses
  A. Airway clearance, ineffective

    B. Breathing pattern, ineffective

    C. Cardiac output, decreased

    D. Fear

    E. Fluid volume deficit

    F. Gas exchange, impaired

    G. Infection, potential for

    H. Injury, potential for

    I. Knowledge deficit related to hazards in the environment

    J. Pain

    K. Poisoning, potential for

    L. Tissue perfusion, altered
- 1. Renal
- 2. Cerebral
- 3. Cardiopulmonary
- 4. Gastrointestinal
- 5. Peripheral

III. Specific environmental emergencies

    A. Thermoregulatory emergencies
- 1. Heat cramps
- 2. Heat exhaustion
- 3. Heat stroke
- 4. Frostbite
- 5. Hypothermia

    B. Near-drowning
- 1. Incidence
- 2. Age of the victim
- 3. Alcohol or drug ingestion
- 4. Freshwater drowning
- 5. Saltwater drowning
- 6. Initial insult: pulmonary
- 7. Secondary insult: pulmonary

    C. Hazardous material incidents
- 1. Source of contamination
- 2. History of exposure
- 3. Decontamination
- 4. Disaster plans
- 5. Medications

    D. Electrical injuries
- 1. Environmental safety
- 2. History of the injury: entrance and exit wounds

3. AC vs. DC current
4. ABCDE: immobilize cervical spine
5. Fluid resuscitation
6. Mannitol and dextran

  E. Lightning injuries

1. History
2. Signs and symptoms
3. Patient outcomes

  F. Burns

1. Sources
   a. Thermal
   b. Chemical
   c. Environmental
2. Depth of the burn
   a. Degree
   b. Skin thickness
3. Extent of the burn
   a. *Rule of Nines*
   b. Lund and Browder Chart
4. Burn treatment
   a. Fluid resuscitation
   b. Treatment of other injuries
   c. Wound care

INTRODUCTION

The environment that surrounds us not only provides us with beauty, but is a source of potential dangers as well. Throughout human evolution, we have learned to adjust to our surroundings. This has been done by controlling our environment. However, there are still forces in the environment that cannot be controlled. In these circumstances humankind has had to learn to live within the environment or suffer the consequences.

To understand the effects of the environment on a patient, one must be familiar with how the body interacts with the environment. Body temperature, or thermoregulation, is maintained by the hypothalamus. The preoptic anterior hypothalamus receives body temperature information from the peripheral and central nervous systems. Several systems interact to help control or "adjust" the body temperature. These include the pituitary and adrenal glands and the sympathetic nervous system. The sympathetic nervous system manages vasodilation and vasoconstriction. In addition, the processes of convection, radiation, and evaporation contribute to the regulation of body temperature.[1]

The initial care of the patient who has suffered an illness or injury from the environment is based on removing the patient from the injurious environment when possible and assuring that the environment in which the caregivers (including the emergency nurse) are to work is safe. The caregivers need to be appropriately dressed; additional hazards such as radiation or chemical toxins need to be contained; and the appropriate authorities need to be notified so that the victim receives the best possible care.

The general management of the patient who has suffered an illness or injury from the environment is based on the initial evaluation and stabilization of the ABCs. It is important to expose the patient. Exposure will help the emergency nurse identify the cause of the problem, as well as any additional injuries. Vital signs, particularly the patient's temperature, should be evaluated.

Obtaining a history of what happened will help the emergency nurse recognize the type of environmental illness or injury the patient has suffered. Information should include the type of environmental surroundings in which the patient was found, any significant exposure to toxins, the length of time the patient was exposed, the patient's previous medical history, current medications, and any recent use of alcohol or drugs. It is important to remember that both the young and the old are at greater risk for suffering injury or illness from the environment.[1]

The initial emergency nursing interventions are based on the specific illness or injury suffered by the patient. Intravenous access will need to be obtained and medications administered as needed. A baseline neurological assessment should be obtained to set the foundation for further assessment and to evaluate the effects of specific treatments. Wound care is initiated in the emergency department. Finally, the appropriate authorities will need to be notified and/or consulted in order to provide additional information for patient care.[1,2]

REVIEW QUESTIONS
Heat-Related Emergencies

An 85-year-old woman is brought to the emergency department. It is a very hot day, with the outside temperature in the 90s and the humidity at 97%. The patient is unconscious; her blood pressure is 90/50; her pulse is 120; her respiratory rate is 28 with shallow respirations; and her rectal temperature is 106° F.

1. The major difference between heat exhaustion and heat stroke is the:

0   A. Patient's level of consciousness
0   B. Fact that the patient with heat exhaustion is hypotensive
0   C. Fact that the patient with heat stroke does not sweat
0   D. Patient's age

2. One of the primary interventions in the care of the patient who is suffering from heat stroke is:
0   A. Rapid cooling
0   B. Insertion of a rectal temperature probe
0   C. Performing a baseline neurological assessment
0   D. Giving the patient oral fluids

3. Based on this patient's blood pressure and pulse, the following is the most appropriate nursing diagnosis:
0   A. Airway clearance, ineffective
0   B. Pain
0   C. Fluid volume deficit
0   D. Breathing pattern, ineffective

4. The patient is being cooled with wet sheets and large fans. During the cooling process, the emergency nurse should frequently evaluate what physiological system for complications?
0   A. Cardiovascular
0   B. Pulmonary
0   C. Renal
0   D. Neurological

•   •   •

5. Drugs that leave a patient at greater risk for developing a heat-related emergency include:
0   A. Narcotics
0   B. Benzodiazepines
0   C. Phenothiazines
0   D. Nonsteroidal antiinflammatory agents

Heat cramps

An 18-year-old man comes to the emergency department complaining of weakness and cramps in his legs. He has been out working with a paving crew. The outside temperature is 90° F, and the humidity is 80%.

6. The major cause of heat cramps is:

   0 A. Fluid retention that causes swelling in the lower extremities

   0 B. Loss of salt in thermal sweat without adequate replacement in oral fluids

   0 C. Hyperventilation tetany that occurs with heat exhaustion

   0 D. Drinking excessive amounts of Gatorade during outside exercise in a hot environment

7. The best treatment for the patient with heat cramps is:

   0 A. Inserting two large-bore IV needles and giving a fluid bolus of normal saline

   0 B. Elevating the extremities that are causing the patient discomfort

   0 C. Oral ingestion of a balanced salt solution

   0 D. Insertion of a nasogastric tube and irrigation with cool saline solution

8. The patient is treated for heat cramps. What nursing diagnosis should the emergency nurse use to base the patient's discharge planning on?

   0 A. Fear related to suddenly being sick

   0 B. Knowledge deficit related to the causes of heat cramps

   0 C. Fluid volume deficit related to the hot environment

   0 D. Self-esteem disturbance related to becoming ill on the job

9. One evaluation criterion the emergency nurse could use to assess whether this patient understood his discharge instructions would be the fact that the patient:

   0 A. States ways to prevent heat cramps

   0 B. Returns the next day with heat cramps

   0 C. Quits his job

   0 D. Returns in a hypernatremic state

Cold-Related Emergencies

10. Superficial frostbite is treated by:

   0 A. Warming the tissue in warm water

   0 B. Rubbing the affected area with snow

   0 C. Covering the affected area with wool

   0 D. Protecting the patient from infection

Hypothermia

A 40-year-old man is brought to the emergency department after having been foundly-ing under a bridge in a sleeping bag. The outside temperature has ranged from 20° to 35° F. No one knows how long the man had been lying there. He is responding only to deep pain. His blood pressure is 100/70; he has a pulse rate of 60 and a respiratory rate of 10. His core body temperature is 85° F.

11. What is the potentially lethal cardiac dysrhythmia associated with the hypothermic patient?
   0   A. Ventricular fibrillation
   0   B. Paroxysmal atrial tachycardia
   0   C. Sinus bradycardia
   0   D. Multifocal premature ventricular contractions (PVCs)

12. What additional laboratory studies would be of value in the initial management of this patient?
   0   A. Aminophylline level
   0   B. Phenytoin level
   0   C. Alcohol level
   0   D. Minoxidil level

13. During the initial rewarming of the hypothermic patient, the most appropriate nursing diagnosis is:
   0   A. Knowledge deficit related to proper dress
   0   B. Pain
   0   C. Injury, potential for
   0   D. Infection, potential for

14. Because of the sludging of blood that can occur in the hypothermic patient, fluid resuscitation will need to be initiated to prevent such complications as acute tubular necrosis. What criteria should the emergency nurse use to evaluate the effectiveness of the fluid resuscitation?
   0   A. Changes in mental status
   0   B. Changes in peripheral pulses
   0   C. Changes in core body temperature
   0   D. Changes in CVP and urinary output

Near-Drowning

A 3-year-old boy is brought to the emergency department after having been found at the bottom of a swimming pool. CPR was initiated by his mother. On arrival in the emergency department, the child is intubated with spontaneous respirations; he has a blood pressure of 80/50 and a pulse of 140.

15. The history obtained about the near-drowning incident should contain all of the following *except* the:

0   A. Age of the victim
0   B. Length of time the victim was under the water
0   C. Temperature of the water
0   D. Age of the patient's mother

16. An important *initial* intervention in the management of the unconscious victim of near-drowning is:
    0   A. Rewarming the patient
    0   B. Immobilization of the cervical spine
    0   C. Drawing blood gases
    0   D. Obtaining a chest x-ray film

17. This child's initial blood gases are pH, 7.25; PO_2, 78; PCO_2, 30; and HCO_3, 25. The most appropriate nursing diagnosis is:
    0   A. Gas exchange, impaired
    0   B. Fluid volume deficit
    0   C. Cardiac output, decreased
    0   D. Tissue perfusion, altered (cerebral)

18. The following is a useful tool for continuous cerebral evaluation of the unconscious near-drowning victim in the emergency department:
    0   A. Ice water calorics
    0   B. Occulocephalic reflex
    0   C. Glasgow Coma Scale
    0   D. Deep tendon reflexes

Burns

A 20-year-old man is brought to the emergency department after having been pulled out of a burning building. He is unconscious and has sustained significant burns to his face, arms, and chest.

19. Signs and symptoms of an inhalation injury include:
    0   A. Singed nasal hair
    0   B. Sooty mucous membranes
    0   C. Stridor
    0   D. All of the above

20. Based on this patient's history, what additional laboratory test should be obtained during his initial evaluation?
    0   A. Hepatic profile

0 B. Carboxyhemoglobin
0 C. Type and screen
0 D. Cardiac enzymes

21. A partial-thickness burn causes injury to:
0   A. Muscles
0   B. Subcutaneous tissues
0   C. Regenerative epithelial cells
0   D. The upper portion of the dermis

22. The burns around this patient's chest are found to be circumferential. Because of this type of injury, the most appropriate nursing diagnosis on which the emergency nurse may base care is:
0   A. Breathing pattern, ineffective
0   B. Fluid volume deficit
0   C. Cardiac output, decreased
0   D. Family processes, altered

23. Using the fluid resuscitation formula (Parkland formula) — 4 ml of Ringer's lactate solution times total body surface area (TBSA) burned times patient's weight in kilograms — how much fluid should this patient receive in the first 8 hours (rounded to the nearest 10 ml)? His body weight is 175 pounds. The amount of body surface burned is 25%.
0   A. 7500 ml
0   B. 3750 ml
0   C. 8000 ml
0   D. 5000 ml

24. Because of the pulmonary injury this patient has suffered, what would be the best evaluative criterion the emergency nurse could use to monitor this patient?
0   A. A capillary refill time greater than 2 seconds
0   B. The patient's ability to cough
0   C. The patient's ventilatory patterns
0   D. The patient's tidal volume

• • •

25. Wound care of a minor burn (partial thickness less than 15% in the adult and less than 10% in the child) would consist of:
0   A. Ice directly on the wound

0   B. Povidone-iodine (Betadine) solution directly on the wound
0   C. Washing with a mild soapy solution
0   D. Rinsing the wound with turpentine

26. What type of ultraviolet radiation causes a sunburn?
   0   A. Ultraviolet C radiation
   0   B. Ultraviolet B radiation
   0   C. Ultraviolet A radiation
   0   D. Ultraviolet D radiation

27. An 18-month-old girl is brought to the emergency department by her parents after having bitten into an electrical cord. The child has a large blister and a charred wound on the right side of her lip. A delayed consequence of this type of burn would be:
   0   A. Cardiac dysrhythmia
   0   B. Hypovolemic shock
   0   C. Bleeding
   0   D. Cataracts

Electrical Injuries

A 30-year-old construction worker is brought to the emergency department by the rescue squad after having sustained an electrical shock of 10,000 volts. On arrival, he is alert and oriented, complaining of tingling in his left foot. His vital signs are blood pressure, 120/70; pulse, 100; and respiratory rate, 18.

28. All of the following factors determine the nature and severity of electrical injuries *except* the:
   0   A. Age of the patient
   0   B. Amperage
   0   C. Type of current
   0   D. Duration of contact with the current

29. During the initial evaluation of this patient, the emergency nurse should assess for:
   0   A. Fractures
   0   B. Entrance and exit wounds
   0   C. Cataracts
   0   D. Psychosis

30. Because of the effects of electricity on the cardiovascular system, the

most appropriate nursing diagnosis that the emergency nurse could use in planning the care of this patient is:

  0   A. Injury, potential for
  0   B. Infection, potential for
  0   C. Fear
  0   D. Cardiac output, decreased

Lightning Injuries

Everyday there are approximately 8,000,000 lightning flashes throughout the world. Between 200 and 300 people are killed each year by lightning strikes. However, 70% to 80% of people struck by lightning survive.[3]

Even though this is not a common environmental emergency seen by the emergency nurse, it is important to be aware of the possibility of a lightning strike occurring no matter where one works. People at risk include campers, golfers, farmers, forest rangers, and construction workers.[3]

31. All of the following are *early* indications that a person may have been struck by lightning *except:*

  0   A. Vaporized rainwater
  0   B. Feathery skin burns
  0   C. A ruptured tympanic membrane
  0   D. Cataracts

32. The initial management of the patient who is suspected of having been struck by lightning includes:

  0   A. Treating the burns with antibiotic ointment and loose dressings
  0   B. Airway management with cervical spine immobilization
  0   C. Inserting two large-bore IV needles for aggressive fluid resuscitation
  0   D. Placing the patient on a cardiac monitor and treating any life-threatening dysrhythmia

Hazardous Materials

A 40-year-old woman is brought to the emergency department after exposure to radiation at a local industry. The patient had fallen and sustained a broken right arm while trying to run out of the room where the radiation leak was found. The patient's skin was initially cleansed with soap and water at the scene.

33. To prepare for the care of this patient, the decontamination area in the emergency department should contain all of the following *except:*

0   A. An open ventilation system
0   B. A separate water-draining system
0   C. Protective clothing for health care providers
0   D. A dosimeter

34. A median lethal dose of radiation exposure for a human is:
0   A. 2400 rad
0   B. 150 rad
0   C. 350 rad
0   D. 50 rad

35. A fireman sustains a chemical burn from hydrofluoric acid to both upper extremities during the control of a hazardous spill from an over-turned tanker. After assessment and stabilization of the ABCs, the initial care of this patient should include:
0   A. Flushing his burns with sodium bicarbonate
0   B. Putting antibiotic ointment on his burns
0   C. Giving the patient tetanus immunization
0   D. Flushing the burns with normal saline

36. In planning nursing care for patients who have been involved in a hazardous spill or radiation exposure, which of the following nursing diagnoses would be most appropriate?
0   A. Injury, potential for, related to environmental hazards
0   B. Fear related to the unknown effects of the environmental hazards
0   C. Suffocation, potential for, related to the environmental hazards
0   D. Spiritual distress (distress of the human spirit) related to potential damage to the environment because of toxic substances

ANSWERS

1. **C. Assessment.** The patient with heat exhaustion and heat stroke may have similar signs and symptoms. Signs and symptoms of these heat-related illnesses include changes in mental status, hypotension, and tachycardia. The patient suffering from heat exhaustion, however, sweats freely and may even complain of chilling.[2]

2. **A. Intervention.** In addition to the initial management of the ABCs, the primary care of the patient with heat stroke includes rapid cooling. There are several methods available for cooling the patient, including using ice packs, wetting the patient down, and using large fans, cold water immersion, and rectal and gastric lavage.[2]

3. **C. Analysis.** Because of the large volume of fluid that has been lost through sweating, the patient with heat stroke will develop hypotension. Defining characteristics of fluid volume deficit include hypotension, tachycardia, dry skin, dry mucous membranes, and decreased skin turgor.[4]

4. **B. Evaluation.** Even though all the patient's systems are affected during the cooling process, the pulmonary system displays the most frequent source of complications. These complications include the potential for aspiration and pulmonary edema.[2]

5. **C. Assessment.** There are several types of drugs that can contribute to a patient being at greater risk for developing heat stroke, including antipsychotics, anticholinergics, tricyclics, and major tranquilizers.[2]

6. **B. Assessment.** Heat cramps are related to the loss of salt in thermal sweat from working in a hot environment. Heat cramps differ from exercise cramps in that they tend to occur while the person is resting and do not resolve spontaneously.[5]

7. **C. Intervention.** Heat cramps are usually treated with oral ingestion of a salt solution. The emergency nurse must also keep in mind that the patient with heat cramps may be hypochloremic. Careful evaluation of all the patient's electrolytes is important.[6]

8. **B. Analysis.** The most appropriate nursing diagnosis on which to base this patient's discharge planning is knowledge deficit related to the causes of heat cramps.

9. **A. Evaluation.** The best criterion to use to evaluate discharge instructions is to have the patient explain the instructions to the emergency nurse.[7]

10. **A. Intervention.** The affected part should be rewarmed in water with a temperature of 105° to 115° F. In addition, the patient's core temperature needs to be monitored for hypothermia.[2]

11. **A. Assessment.** When the patient's core body temperature is below 86° F, he or she is at greater risk of developing ventricular fibrillation. This dysrhythmia can be easily stimulated by such procedures as the insertion of monitoring lines. At temperatures between 82.4° and 86° F, ventricular fibrillation may not respond to drugs or countershock.[2]

12. **C. Intervention.** The patient who is intoxicated is at greater risk of developing hypothermia. Alcohol will dull the patient's response to the cold, as well as cause vasodilation and increase the rapidity of heat loss.[2]

13. **C. Analysis.** During the rewarming process the patient is at great risk of being injured. Sources of injury include the rewarming process, the risk of developing seizures during rewarming interventions, and the risk of aspiration.[4]

14. **D. Evaluation.** Fluid resuscitation is best monitored by changes in the

patient's CVP (central venous pressure) and urinary output. These parameters help prevent the possibility of fluid overload.

15. **D. Assessment.** Factors that affect the outcome of a near-drowning victim include the age of the victim, the amount of time spent immersed in the liquid, the development of hypothermia, and the immediacy of resuscitative efforts.[2]

16. **B. Intervention.** The cervical spine should be immobilized in the unconscious near-drowning victim until possible injury to the cervical spine can be evaluated. The child was initially found unconscious at the bottom of the pool. He could have fallen into the pool or struck his head on the bottom of the pool.

17. **A. Analysis.** The defining characteristics of impaired gas exchange include hypercapnia and hypoxia. Because of the aspiration of water, the child's lungs have sustained an alteration in alveolar capillary membrane function.[4,8]

18. **C. Evaluation.** The Glasgow Coma Scale can be a useful tool for ongoing evaluation of cerebral function of the near-drowning victim. The coma scale includes verbal response, eye opening, and motor response.[2]

19. **D. Assessment.** All of the above are signs and symptoms of inhalation injury. In addition, the patient may have other signs and symptoms, including hoarseness, circumoral burns, and restlessness.[3]

20. **B. Intervention.** Because the patient was potentially involved in an enclosed space and because he is unconscious, a carboxyhemoglobin level should be obtained so that the patient can be evaluated for carbon monoxide poisoning. Carbon monoxide will bind with hemoglobin 240 times faster than will oxygen, causing the patient to become hypoxic.[7]

21. **D. Assessment.** Partial-thickness, or second-degree, burns cause injury to the upper portion of the dermis. First-degree burns cause injury to the epidermal layer of the skin. Full-thickness, or third-degree, burns cause injury through the epidermis, dermis, subcutaneous tissues, and muscles. These burns will damage the regenerative epithelial cells, destroy nerve endings, and cause vessel thrombosis.[7]

22. **A. Analysis.** Circumferential burns of the body—particularly the chest and neck—can impair respiratory function. A defining characteristic of this nursing diagnosis is altered chest excursion. Because of the constriction caused by the burn injury, the patient cannot ventilate properly.[4,7]

23. **B. Intervention.** This calculation would be:

$$4 \text{ ml} \times 25 \times 75 = 7500 \text{ ml}$$

One half of this should be given in the first 8 hours. That would be 3750 ml.

24. **C. Evaluation.** The most useful evaluative criterion for this patient would be his ventilatory patterns. Since this patient is at risk for ventilation problems from circumferential burns and for hypoxia from inhalation injury and carbon dioxide poisoning, the pattern of his ventilatory efforts will need to be closely monitored.

25. **C. Intervention.** Ice or povidone-iodine (Betadine) directly on the wound would only cause additional damage to the skin. The skin is the largest organ system, and when it is intact, it prevents toxins from entering the body, in addition to regulating body temperature. When it has been damaged, as in a burn injury, these functions are compromised. Washing with mild soap will help remove any debris from the burn and help prevent infection.[6]

26. **B. Assessment.** Ultraviolet B waves are the main cause of sunburn and skin cancer.[6]

27. **C. Assessment.** A delayed complication of this type of burn would be bleeding. The labial arteries can begin bleeding 3 to 5 days after the injury. The emergency nurse will need to teach the parents to use direct pressure to control the bleeding and return the child for further evaluation if the bleeding does not stop.[9]

28. **A. Assessment.** There are six major factors that determine the nature and severity of an electrical injury: voltage, amperage, type of current, duration of contact, current path through the victim, and skin resistance.[10]

29. **B. Assessment.** Locating the entrance and exit wounds through which the electricity passed will help the emergency nurse determine which path the current traveled on. Effects from electrical current passage may interfere with the cardiac, respiratory, and neurological systems.[2]

30. **D. Analysis.** Because of the effects of electricity on the cardiovascular system, close monitoring of the cardiovascular system is important. Defining characteristics of this nursing diagnosis include dysrhythmia, ECG changes, hypotension, cold, clammy skin, and variations in hemodynamic readings.[4]

31. **D. Assessment.** Cataracts are a late sign of injury from a lightning strike. Four types of injuries initially occur after a lightning strike: cardiac injuries, neurological injuries, burns, and blunt trauma.[3]

32. **B. Intervention.** Many times when patients are struck by lightning, they are found to be apneic. Because of the possibility of cervical spine trauma, the patient's airway needs to be approached with cervical spine immobilization.[3,6]

33. **A. Intervention.** Emergency department preparedness for the victim of radiation exposure should include a formal policy concerning the equip-

ment and care of the patient who has suffered exposure to radiation, protective gear for health care providers, a separate drainage system for water, and a dosimeter to measure the amount of exposure health care providers may be subjected to.[11]

34. **C. Assessment.** Fifty percent of humans who are exposed to 350 rad will die of radiation poisoning.[12]

35. **D. Intervention.** Chemical burns should be flushed with copious amounts of water or normal saline.[13]

36. **A. Analysis.** Injury, potential for, would be the most appropriate nursing diagnosis and includes individual(s) at risk of injury from environmental sources, such as pollutants, poisons, physical design of the environment, and improperly used equipment.[14]

REFERENCES

1. Sollars G: Thermoregulatory emergencies. In Kitt S, Kaiser J, editors: *Emergency nursing: a physiologic and clinical perspective*, Philadelphia, 1990, WB Saunders.
2. Stewart C: *Environmental emergencies*, Baltimore, 1990, Williams & Wilkins.
3. Woolley S, Druek C: Burn injuries. In Kitt S, Kaiser J, editors: *Emergency nursing: a physiologic and clinical perspective*, Philadelphia, 1990, WB Saunders.
4. McFarland GK, McFarlane EA: *Nursing diagnosis and intervention: planning for patient care*, St Louis, 1989, Mosby–Year Book.
5. Auerbach PS, Geehr EC: *Management of wilderness and environmental emergencies*, ed 2, St Louis, 1989, Mosby–Year Book.
6. Trott A: *Minor wound care*, New York, 1985, Medical Examination Publishing.
7. Carlson JH et al: *Nursing diagnosis: a case study approach*, Philadelphia, 1991, WB Saunders.
8. Goldman M: Pediatric medical emergencies. In Kitt S, Kaiser J, editors: *Emergency nursing: a physiologic and clinical perspective*, Philadelphia, 1990, WB Saunders.
9. Cole JA, Plantz SH: *Emergency medicine*, New York, 1990, McGraw-Hill.
10. Fontanarosa P: Lightning and related injuries, *J Emerg Med Serv* 13(7):37-43, 1988.
11. Tortella BJ: Risks to the emergency medical service provider: radiation, the EMS environment, and the combative patient, *Emerg Care Q* 5(4):40-47.
12. Thomas HA, O'Connor R, Hoffman G: *Emergency medicine: self-assessment and review*, ed 2, St Louis, 1988, Mosby–Year Book.
13. Sheehy SB: *Mosby's manual of emergency care*, ed 3, St Louis, 1990, Mosby–Year Book.
14. Carlson JH et al: *Nursing diagnosis: a case study approach*, Philadelphia, 1991, WB Saunders.

Chapter 5
Facial Emergencies

REVIEW OUTLINE

I.   Anatomy and physiology
   A. Anatomical structures
      1. Mandible
      2. Maxilla
      3. Zygoma
      4. Zygomatic arch
      5. Nasal bones and structures
      6. Orbit
      7. Orbital rim
      8. Sinuses
        a. Frontal
        b. Maxillary
        c. Ethmoid
        d. Sphenoid
      9. Ethmoid bone
     10. Cranial nerves
     11. Cranial bones
     12. Oral cavity and contents
     13. Auditory bones and structures
     14. Major blood vessels
   B. Physiology
      1. Central nervous system
        a. Cranial nerves
        b. Functions of brainstem, cerebrum, and cerebellum
      2. Process of sight
      3. Process of speech

II. Assessment
    A. Primary survey
        1. ABCDE (airway, breathing, circulation, deficit [neurological], exposure)
        2. Stabilization
    B. Secondary survey
        1. History of illness or injury
            a. Mechanism and time
            b. AMPLE history
                (1) Allergies
                (2) Medications
                (3) Past medical history
                (4) Last meal
                (5) Events or treatment prior to arrival
        2. Chief complaint
            a. Pain: PQRST
                (1) Provocation
                (2) Quality
                (3) Radiation
                (4) Severity
                (5) Timing
            b. Bleeding
            c. Edema, ecchymosis
            d. Asymmetry
            e. Fever, chills
            f. Paresthesia
            g. Diplopia
            h. Malocclusion
            i. Trismus
            j. Deformity
        3. Physical examination
            a. General appearance
            b. Mental status, level of consciousness
            c. Glasgow Coma Scale score
            d. Vital signs
            e. Inspection
                (1) Symmetry of facial features
                (2) Ecchymosis
                (3) Edema
                (4) Eyes: subconjunctival hemorrhage, pupillary height, pupillary reaction, extraocular eye movements (EOMs)

(5) Nose
(6) Mouth, malocclusion
(7) Ears
(8) Cranial nerves
(9) Scalp
(10) Neck
(11) Head
f. Palpation
(1) Symmetry
(2) Localized point tenderness
(3) Abnormal mobility
(4) Crepitus
(5) Temporomandibular joint (TMJ)
(6) Foreign bodies
(7) Lacerations, hematomas
III. Diagnostic studies or procedures
A. Radiology
B. Laboratory
IV. Related nursing diagnoses
A. Airway clearance, ineffective
B. Anxiety
C. Fluid volume deficit (actual or potential)
D. Infection, potential for
E. Knowledge deficit
F. Pain
G. Sensory/perceptual alterations
H. Skin integrity, impaired

INTRODUCTION

Maxillofacial emergencies are common in any emergency department. Most injuries are not life threatening, but the potential for disfigurement and emotional despair is great. The most common mechanism of injury producing facial injuries is blunt trauma secondary to motor vehicle accidents. Other mechanisms of injury include those that produce both blunt and penetrating trauma, such as altercations, domestic violence, falls, and sports-related accidents.

Maxillofacial emergencies produce life-threatening situations through their ability to obstruct the airway and cause hemorrhagic shock. Mechanical obstruction of the airway occurs as a result of anatomical displacement of normal structures secondary to trauma or disease. Broken teeth or a swollen epiglottis are examples of such. Because the head in general is rich in vasculature, profuse bleeding is a natural occurrence with any injury. Maxillofacial trauma can cause severe hemorrhage, which may be occult, since patients have a tendency to swallow blood rather than expectorate it.

Assessment and stabilization of clients with maxillofacial emergencies follow the same sequence, the ABCs, as for any trauma patient.

REVIEW QUESTIONS
Facial Trauma

A 26-year-old woman is brought to the emergency department by the rescue squad. She was the unrestrained driver of an automobile that ran into a bridge abutment. The car's windshield was reportedly cracked. The victim, Ms. Green, is awake and oriented. A large scalp laceration and facial trauma are obvious. Ms. Green's vital signs are blood pressure, 90/60; pulse, 100; and respiratory rate, 28. Ms. Green has been appropriately immobilized on a backboard with a cervical collar in place.

1. The first priority in the assessment of this patient is:
   - 0   A. Airway
   - 0   B. Breathing
   - 0   C. Circulation
   - 0   D. Deficit (neurological)

2. The most appropriate method for assessment of Ms. Green's airway would be to:
   - 0   A. Auscultate the chest for normal breath sounds
   - 0   B. Ask the patient if she is getting enough air
   - 0   C. Have Ms. Green open her mouth and observe for foreign bodies
   - 0   D. Draw arterial blood gases to evaluate oxygen saturation

3. When assessing Ms. Green's airway, the nurse discovers that the patient has a large amount of bleeding into the oropharynx, which she is swallowing. The immediate intervention should be to:
   - 0   A. Wait until the cervical spine is cleared and then place the patient in a semi-Fowler's position
   - 0   B. Perform frequent suctioning and teach the patient to expectorate the blood
   - 0   C. Prepare for intubation to protect the airway
   - 0   D. Insert a nasogastric tube to withdraw the swallowed blood

4. Based on the mechanism of injury and Ms. Green's vital signs, the most appropriate nursing diagnosis is:
0   A. Grieving, anticipatory
0   B. Hyperthermia
0   C. Fluid volume deficit
0   D. Thought processes, altered

Ms. Green is diagnosed as having a bilateral LeForte III fracture, also known as "craniofacial dysjunction." As its name implies, the facial and cranial skulls become disjoined in this type of fracture. A LeForte I fracture produces a horizontal detachment of the maxilla at the level of the nasal floor, leaving the maxillary alveolar ridge and hard palate mobile. A LeForte II, or "pyramid fracture," involves fractures of the maxilla, nasal bones, the medial half of the interior orbital rim, the orbital floor, and lacrimal bones.

5. A common emergency nursing intervention is to monitor airway patency. What criterion is the first indicator of airway compromise?
0   A. Change in respiratory rate
0   B. Change in color
0   C. Change in mental status
0   D. Change in blood pressure and pulse

Blowout Fractures

Mr. Plant, a 32-year-old man, is brought to the emergency department by the police after his involvement in an altercation. He has sustained facial trauma and is diagnosed as having a blowout orbital fracture on the right. He is awake and alert with no other obvious injuries. Mr. Plant's vital signs are blood pressure, 120/80; pulse, 84; and respiratory rate, 18.

6. Common signs and symptoms of a blowout orbital fracture include:
0   A. Blindness on the affected side
0   B. A flattened cheek on the affected side
0   C. Lowered pupil position on the affected side
0   D. Extraocular eye movements limited bilaterally

7. The most appropriate nursing diagnosis for Mr. Plant would be:
0   A. Thought processes, altered
0   B. Hopelessness
0   C. Fluid volume deficit
0   D. Pain

8. An appropriate nursing intervention related to the above nursing diagnosis would be to:
   - 0 A. Apply ice
   - 0 B. Administer analgesics as ordered
   - 0 C. Assist the patient to a semi-Fowler's position after his cervical spine has been cleared
   - 0 D. All of the above

   • • •

9. The patient who has sustained a blowout orbital fracture and has periorbital emphysema should have his or her visual acuity monitored to evaluate for involvement of the:
   - 0 A. Central retinal artery
   - 0 B. Extraocular eye muscles
   - 0 C. Intraorbital nerves
   - 0 D. Optic nerve

10. If the patient with periorbital emphysema complains of a sudden decrease in visual acuity, the nurse should:
    - 0 A. Prepare for immediate surgery
    - 0 B. Reassess the patient's visual acuity
    - 0 C. Prepare for a lateral canthotomy or intraorbital needle aspiration
    - 0 D. Have the patient lie flat and turn on the unaffected side

Bell's Palsy

Mrs. Jones, a 45-year-old woman, comes to the emergency department with peripheral facial paralysis, fever, chills, and flulike symptoms. She is diagnosed as having Bell's palsy. This is Mrs. Jones's first episode of any type of disorder, and she is very anxious.

11. Bell's palsy affects which cranial nerve?
    - 0 A. Fourth: trochlear
    - 0 B. Fifth: trigeminal
    - 0 C. Seventh: facial
    - 0 D. Ninth: glossopharyngeal

12. Common signs and symptoms associated with Bell's palsy include:
    - 0 A. Onset of symptoms occurs gradually
    - 0 B. Increased lacrimation on the affected side
    - 0 C. Unilateral, flaccid facial paralysis
    - 0 D. Lid lag on the opposite side, especially noted when closing the eyes

13. The most appropriate nursing diagnosis for Mrs. Jones is:

   0   A. Anxiety related to knowledge deficit

   0   B. Airway clearance, ineffective

   0   C. Hopelessness

   0   D. Infection, potential for

14. The most appropriate nursing intervention related to the above nursing diagnosis involves education. Mrs. Jones should be taught that:

   0   A. She must be admitted to the hospital to rule out a cerebrovascular accident (CVA)

   0   B. Recovery is usually spontaneous and occurs within 3 weeks

   0   C. To facilitate recovery, she must enter a rehabilitation program immediately

   0   D. She will never recover and must learn to live with permanent Bell's phenomenon

15. Mrs. Jones is very upset and wants to know what caused this. The nurse's most appropriate reply would be:

   0   A. Herpes simplex

   0   B. Emotional stress

   0   C. Prolonged exposure to drafts and/or cold

   0   D. All of the above

Infection

A 10-year-old boy, Tommy, is brought to the emergency department by his mother after his involvement in a bicycle accident. Tommy fell head first on a gravel road. He was not unconscious; on arrival in the emergency department he is awake and oriented. He has sustained a deep facial laceration extending from the forehead through the left eyebrow. He also has multiple facial abrasions. His vital signs are stable, and he has no other obvious injuries.

16. Assessment of all the wounds for the presence of foreign bodies is imperative to prevent:

   0   A. Potential infection

   0   B. Potential "tattooing" effect

   0   C. Improper wound closure (malalignment)

   0   D. All of the above

17. The primary nursing diagnosis related to Tommy's mechanism of injury is:

   0   A. Infection, potential for

0   B. Body temperature, altered, potential
0   C. Gas exchange, impaired
0   D. Fluid volume deficit

18. Preparation of Tommy's large laceration for suturing includes all of the following except:
    0   A. Anesthesizing the wound prior to cleansing
    0   B. Shaving the eyebrow to remove all surrounding debris
    0   C. Cleansing with the appropriate solution and rinsing thoroughly
    0   D. Searching thoroughly for foreign bodies with a magnification instrument (glasses or lens)

19. Tommy's mother is taught to observe for signs of infection. To evaluate the effectiveness of education, the emergency nurse should:
    0   A. Have Tommy's mother repeat what she has been taught
    0   B. Make an appointment for Tommy to return to the emergency department for a wound check
    0   C. Call Tommy's pediatrician the next day to make sure Tommy's mother has made an appointment for a wound check and suture removal
    0   D. Make a written referral to the local public health department requesting follow-up information on Tommy

ANSWERS

1. **A. Assessment.** Obviously, the patient cannot survive without a patent airway. All other assessment parameters are secondary to airway assessment.
2. **C. Assessment.** This is the best method for assessing Ms. Green's airway because of the potential for foreign bodies. The most common foreign bodies seen in maxillofacial trauma are broken teeth, the tongue, and blood. The tongue may obstruct the airway in patients with a decreased level of consciousness. It is important to actively look for broken teeth and the amount of occult bleeding, since fearful patients can easily hide both.
3. **B. Intervention.** Waiting until the cervical spine is cleared and then repositioning the patient may be too late. Frequently the swallowed blood produces nausea and vomiting, which further adds to the potential for airway compromise. Intubation is not necessary unless the airway cannot be protected by simple techniques such as suctioning and eventually repositioning. A nasogastric tube may precipitate vomiting.

4. **C. Analysis.** Ms. Green's blood pressure is low and her pulse is above average for the normal adult. Both are signs of hypovolemia.

5. **C. Evaluation.** A change in vital signs is a very late indicator of respiratory compromise. Color is a poor assessment parameter in the adult. Frequently, patients will exhibit very subtle changes in mental status, such as sudden anger, complaints, or sleepiness that the alert emergency nurse must be aware of to provide rapid diagnosis and intervention.

6. **C. Assessment.** A blowout orbital fracture is a depressed fracture of the orbital floor in which the contents of the orbit protrude into the maxillary sinus. Thus the affected eye sinks into the maxillary sinus, producing a lowered pupil position and asymmetry of the eyes on visual inspection of the patient. Other common signs and symptoms of a blowout orbital fracture include conjunctival hemorrhage and eyelid ecchymosis due to blunt trauma, infraorbital nerve paresthesia due to a pinched facial nerve at the fracture site, and diplopia.

7. **D. Analysis.** Blowout orbital fractures alone do not produce impaired thought processes, hopelessness, or fluid volume deficit. They do, however, produce severe pain.

8. **D. Intervention.** Application of ice and elevation of the head will decrease edema, as well as pain. The administration of analgesics will also address the nursing diagnosis of pain.

9. **A. Evaluation.** Air may build up under pressure in the orbit, producing cessation of blood flow in the central retinal artery.

10. **C. Intervention.** This is a true emergent procedure that must be performed in order to save the patient's sight by removing the trapped air.

11. **C. Assessment.**

12. **C. Assessment.** Other signs and symptoms of Bell's palsy include rapid onset of symptoms, viral prodrome, lid lag on the affected side when closing the eyes, decreased lacrimation on the affected side, and Bell's phenomenon, which is an upward movement of the eyeball on the affected side when attempting to close the eye.

13. **A. Analysis.** Bell's palsy does not affect the airway or have the potential for the patient to develop an infectious process. Most patients are extremely anxious because of a lack of knowledge concerning their medical diagnosis.

14. **B. Intervention.** During the recovery phase Mrs. Jones should also be taught to rest and treat her flulike symptoms appropriately. She will also be given eye drops because of the decreased lacrimation on the affected side and may require analgesics.

15. **D. Intervention.** The exact cause of Bell's palsy is unknown, but the

theoretical causes include herpes simplex, emotional stress, and prolonged exposure to drafts and/or cold.

16. **D. Assessment.** Infection, tattooing, and malalignment may result from a missed foreign body.

17. **A. Analysis.** Because Tommy sustained his injury on a gravel road, his potential for infection is high.

18. **B. Intervention.** Eyebrows should never be shaved, since they provide anatomical landmarks to be used to ensure proper alignment of the wound, and they may not grow back.

19. **A. Evaluation.** A return demonstration or repeat of verbal and/or written instructions is the best way to evaluate patient learning.

ADDITIONAL READINGS

Boyne PJ: Early treatment of facial trauma, *Postgrad Med* 11(5):99-111, 1985.

Cantrill SV: Facial trauma and epistaxis. In Rosen P et al, editors: *Emergency medicine: concepts and clinical practice,* ed 2, St Louis, 1988, Mosby–Year Book.

Cantrill SV: Facial trauma. In Barkin RM, Rosen P, editors: *Emergency pediatrics: a guide to ambulatory care,* St Louis, 1990, Mosby–Year Book.

Gerlock AJ: Facial trauma, *Trauma Q* 2(4):20-34, 1986.

Goldman R: For your eyes only, *Emergency* 19(12):27-29, 1987.

Gussack GS et al: Pediatric maxillofacial trauma: unique features in diagnosis and treatment, *Laryngoscope* 97:925-930, 1987.

Kalish MA: Airway management in maxillofacial trauma, *Emerg Med Serv* 18(6):42-44, 1989.

Karesh JW: Ocular and periocular trauma, *Emerg Med Serv* 18(6):46-55, 1989.

Lower J: Maxillofacial trauma, *Nurs Clin North Am* 21(4):611-628, 1986.

Manson PN, Kelly KJ: Evaluation and management of the patient with facial trauma, *Emerg Med Serv* 18(6):22-30, 1989.

Chapter 6
Medical Emergencies

REVIEW OUTLINE
I. Anatomy
   A. Liver
   B. Kidneys
   C. Pancreas
   D. Cerebral cortex
   E. Brainstem
   F. Red blood cells (RBCs)
   G. White blood cells (WBCs)
II. Physiology
   A. Fluid and electrolyte balance
   B. Renin-angiotensin-aldosterone system
   C. Acid-base balance
   D. Renal function
   E. Hepatic function
   F. Glucose metabolism
   G. Clotting mechanisms
   H. Immunity
   I. Inflammatory response
III. Assessment of the patient with a medical emergency
   A. Airway
   B. Breathing-ventilatory patterns
      1. Apnea
      2. Hyperventilation
      3. Cheyne-Stokes respirations
      4. Hypoventilation
      5. Central neurogenic hyperventilation
   C. Circulation
      1. Heart rate, cardiac monitor

  2. Skin color
  3. Skin temperature
  4. Capillary refill
  5. Skin turgor
D. Neurological assessment
  1. Level of consciousness
  2. Pupillary response
  3. Sensory response
  4. Motor response
  5. Oculocephalic reflex
  6. Oculovestibular reflex
  7. Corneal reflex
  8. Decorticate posturing
  9. Decerebrate posturing
  10. Flaccidity
E. History related to the medical emergency
  1. Onset of symptoms
  2. Past medical history
  3. Medications
  4. Allergies
  5. Family/psychosocial history
IV. Collaborative care of the patient with a medical emergency
A. Stabilization of airway, breathing, and circulation
B. Diagnostic studies or procedures
  1. Laboratory tests
    a. Complete blood cell count (CBC)
    b. Electrolytes
    c. Ethanol level
    d. Glucose
    e. Creatinine, blood urea nitrogen (BUN)
    f. Urinalysis
    g. Drug screen
    h. Liver enzymes
    i. Clotting studies
    j. Carboxyhemoglobin
    k. Type and crossmatch
    l. Serum uric acid
    m. Serum ammonia
    n. Reticulocyte count
    o. Cultures

2. ECG
3. Chest x-ray film
4. Arteriogram
5. Doppler studies
6. Ultrasound
7. Computed tomography (CT) scan
8. Magnetic resonance imaging (MRI)

C. Medications
1. Dextrose 50% (D_{50})
2. Naloxone
3. Thiamine
4. Oxygen
5. Antipyretics
6. Probenecid
7. Sulfinpyrazone
8. Colchicine
9. Indomethacin
10. Cryoprecipitate
11. Calcium chloride
12. Insulin
13. Sodium polystyrene sulfonate (Kayexalate)
14. $NaHCO_3$
15. Potassium
16. Antibiotics

V. Related nursing diagnoses
A. Airway clearance, ineffective
B. Aspiration, potential for
C. Body temperature, altered, potential
D. Breathing pattern, ineffective
E. Cardiac output, decreased
F. Diarrhea
G. Fatigue
H. Fluid volume deficit
I. Fluid volume excess
J. Gas exchange, impaired
K. Infection, potential for
L. Injury, potential for
M. Knowledge deficit
N. Pain

VI. Specific medical emergencies

A. Coma
B. Reye's syndrome
C. Gout
D. Sickle cell crisis
E. Hemophilia
F. Dehydration
G. Hepatitis
H. Pancreatitis
I. Fever
J. Acquired immune deficiency syndrome (AIDS)
K. Allergic reaction, anaphylaxis
L. Ketoacidosis
   1. Diabetic
   2. Alcoholic
M. Hyperglycemic hyperosmolar nonketotic coma (HHNC)
N. Meningitis
O. Hyperkalemia
P. Hypokalemia
Q. Hypernatremia
R. Hyponatremia
S. Hypercalcemia
T. Hypocalcemia
U. Transplant recipients
   1. Heart
   2. Kidney
   3. Heart-lung

INTRODUCTION

*M*edical emergencies may not be as dramatic as a cardiac arrest or multiple trauma, but they certainly can be as life threatening. They may present as a cluster of symptoms involving virtually every bodily system. Many medical conditions overlap with or result in other clinical problems. For example, a patient with sickle cell crisis may also have dehydration, fever, and an electrolyte imbalance. Determining the initial presenting problem vs. the ensuing complications is crucial.

People who have emergent medical problems make up a large percentage of the emergency department clientele. As with any other patient, patients with medical emergencies need immediate assessment and stabilization of their airway, breathing, and circulation. The emergency nurse needs to have a thorough understanding of the anatomy and physiology of the involved system(s). A complete history needs to be obtained, along with a complete assessment of the patient's physical state.

The cause of the medical crisis may sometimes be as important as the treatment. The emergency nurse is responsible for coordinating the necessary diagnostic procedures and instituting the appropriate therapy.

REVIEW QUESTIONS
Coma

Mr. Black, a 58-year-old man, is brought to the emergency department one morning after his wife could not awaken him. On arrival he is in a deep coma. His vital signs are blood pressure, 140/92; pulse, 100; and respiratory rate, 36 and irregular.

1. The first priority is to:
   0   A. Determine if any injury has occurred
   0   B. Maintain a patent airway
   0   C. Draw arterial blood gases
   0   D. Arrange for an emergency CT scan of the head

2. Additional assessment and treatment modalities will probably include:
   0   A. Administration of thiamine and dexamethasone (Decadron)
   0   B. A 12-lead ECG and a nonrebreather mask
   0   C. Administration of dextrose 50% IV and naloxone (Narcan) IV
   0   D. Serum and urine drug screens

3. Mr. Black's respiratory pattern is as follows: four rapid deep breaths followed by apnea; then the cycle repeats itself. This is known as:
   0   A. Cheyne-Stokes respirations
   0   B. Central neurogenic hyperventilation
   0   C. Kussmaul's respirations
   0   D. Biot's respirations or cluster breathing

•   •   •

4. The Glasgow Coma Scale measures these three components:
   0   A. Eye movements, verbal response, and motor response
   0   B. Vital signs, sensory/motor function, and pupil reaction
   0   C. Level of consciousness, vital signs, and sensory functions
   0   D. Decorticate, decerebrate, and abnormal posturings

5. The maintenance of brain function mainly requires these two substances:
  0   A. Sodium and potassium
  0   B. DNA and RNA
  0   C. Calcium and magnesium
  0   D. Oxygen and glucose

Joint Pain

6. A patient who has gout (hyperuricemia) is also at greater risk for developing:
  0   A. Myocardial infarction
  0   B. Stroke
  0   C. Renal calculi
  0   D. Sepsis

7. An appropriate nursing diagnosis for a patient with arthritis would be:
  0   A. Pain
  0   B. Cardiac output, decreased
  0   C. Infection, potential for
  0   D. Airway clearance, ineffective

8. A patient with inflammatory joint pain is given a prescription for a non-steroidal antiinflammatory drug (NSAID). It is crucial that the dosage instructions include:
  0   A. "Take this medicine on an empty stomach."
  0   B. "Take this medicine with food or milk."
  0   C. "Never take this medicine with any juices."
  0   D. "Notify your doctor if this medicine makes you nauseated."

9. Classic symptoms of inflammatory joint disease include all of the following *except:*
  0   A. Stiffness and decreased range of motion
  0   B. Erythema and edema
  0   C. Low-grade temperature and fatigue
  0   D. Crepitus and deformity

Sickle Cell Crisis

Mr. Baker, a 24-year-old black man, comes to the emergency department with sickle cell crisis.

10. Symptoms related to sickle cell crisis include all of the following *except:*

0   A. Abdominal, back, and joint pain
0   B. Weakness
0   C. Fever
0   D. Projectile vomiting

11. Primary, initial interventions of sickle cell crisis center mainly around:
0   A. Patient teaching
0   B. Hydration
0   C. Prevention of infection
0   D. Transfusion therapy

12. Complications of untreated sickle cell crisis include:
0   A. Major organ and tissue damage
0   B. Tissue necrosis
0   C. Hemolytic anemia
0   D. All of the above

13. The nurse may be able to identify when Mr. Baker's sickling crisis is over because the:
0   A. Pain subsides and fever decreases
0   B. Urine output is greater than 30 ml/hr
0   C. Heart rate returns to normal
0   D. Hemoglobin level is greater than 10

14. A frequently encountered problem with patients who suffer frequent episodes of sickle cell crisis is:
0   A. Septic shock
0   B. Eventual paralysis
0   C. Narcotic dependency or addiction
0   D. Disseminated intravascular coagulation (DIC)

Dehydration

Mrs. Clark is a 94-year-old patient admitted to the emergency department from a nursing home. She appears to be dehydrated in addition to having a urinary tract infection.

15. Characteristics of dehydration include all of the following *except:*
0   A. Nausea, vomiting, and diarrhea
0   B. Fatigue and muscle cramps
0   C. Fever
0   D. Exophthalmos

16. Laboratory evaluation of dehydration would reveal:
- 0   A. Low hematocrit
- 0   B. Elevated BUN
- 0   C. Serum osmolality of less than 200
- 0   D. Normal BUN

17. The nursing diagnosis for Mrs. Clark would center around:
- 0   A. Fluid volume deficit
- 0   B. Gas exchange, impaired
- 0   C. Tissue integrity, impaired
- 0   D. Urinary elimination, altered patterns

18. Isotonic IV fluid replacement is started. What clinical findings would indicate *inappropriate* fluid therapy?
- 0   A. Bilateral rales
- 0   B. Urine output greater than 30 ml/hr
- 0   C. A decrease in hemoglobin
- 0   D. Central venous pressure (CVP) of 5 cm H_2O

19. If Mrs. Clark develops pulmonary edema, it may initially be treated by:
- 0   A. Furosemide, IV push
- 0   B. Insertion of a Swan-Ganz catheter
- 0   C. Decreasing the IV fluid rate and giving oxygen
- 0   D. Monitoring vital signs and an ECG

Hemophilia

Barry, an 11-year-old boy with hemophilia, is brought to the emergency depart-ment with a 2 cm stab wound to the right side of his chest after falling on a screwdriver.

20. The immediate priority for Barry is to:
- 0   A. Begin arranging transfer to the area's pediatric hospital
- 0   B. Obtain stat lab work to assess clotting capabilities
- 0   C. Immediately administer cryoprecipitate
- 0   D. Maintain airway and ventilation functions

21. Hemophilia is a hereditary blood disorder characterized by a variant form of:
- 0   A. Factor II
- 0   B. Factor VIII

0   C. Prothrombin

0   D. Fibrinogen

22. The wound turns out to be superficial, and minor suturing is all that is required. However, after his wound is sutured, Barry should:

0   A. Be observed for 4 hours for any further bleeding

0   B. Receive 1 unit of cryoprecipitate prophylactically

0   C. Not receive a tetanus toxoid injection

0   D. Be discharged with instructions given to his mother to return if the bleeding worsens

23. Barry's mother tells the nurse that she periodically gives Barry aspirin for joint aches. A nursing diagnosis for Barry's mother would be:

0   A. Knowledge deficit: therapeutic regimen

0   B. Ineffective coping, family

0   C. Injury, potential for

0   D. None; ASA is the drug of choice for a hemophiliac patient with joint pain

24. If Barry were found to be in hypovolemic shock, his therapy would include:

0   A. IV fluids only

0   B. IV fluids and cryoprecipitate

0   C. IV fluids and vitamin K

0   D. None of the above

Fever

25. Symptoms commonly associated with fever include all of the following *except:*

0   A. Appendicitis

0   B. Meningitis

0   C. Congestive heart failure

0   D. Pelvic inflammatory disease (PID)

26. In the elderly, the cause of fever can best be determined by which of the following diagnostic tests?

0   A. Amylase

0   B. Chest x-ray film

0   C. ECG

0   D. CT scan

27. In children, a great concern is that the fever may lead to:
 0   A. Febrile seizures
 0   B. Epilepsy
 0   C. Meningitis
 0   D. Cardiac arrest

28. Basic nursing interventions for a patient with a fever may include all of the following *except:*
 0   A. Culture of actual or potential sources
 0   B. IV fluids
 0   C. Antipyretic and/or antibiotic administration
 0   D. Blankets to prevent chilling

29. After follow-up instructions are given to the parents of a febrile child, which of the following statements would indicate a knowledge deficit on the part of the parents?
 0   A. "We are to bring him back to the emergency room or call our pediatrician if his temperature goes back up."
 0   B. "If his fever returns, we're to give him aspirin either by mouth or suppository."
 0   C. "He can have about anything he wants to drink."
 0   D. "If he doesn't get better in the next 24 to 48 hours, we need to see the doctor."

Communicable Diseases

30. A major concern in men with parotiditis (mumps) is:
 0   A. Gynecomastia
 0   B. Impotence
 0   C. Orchiditis resulting in sterility
 0   D. Oophoritis

31. Pertussis (whooping cough) is found predominantly in infants and children up to age 4. The most likely factor contributing to this increased incidence is:
 0   A. Failure to have the child properly immunized
 0   B. *Haemophilus influenzae*
 0   C. Environmental pollutants
 0   D. Aspirin misuse

32. Rubella is particularly dangerous to pregnant women (both patients and nurses), especially during:

0   A. The first trimester
0   B. The second trimester
0   C. The third trimester
0   D. All of the above

33. Varicella (chickenpox) in young children usually begins with vesicular eruptions on the:
0   A. Perineum and buttocks
0   B. Head and limbs
0   C. Back and chest
0   D. There is no specific sequence or area

34. Infectious mononucleosis ("mono" or "kissing disease") is a contagious illness caused by:
0   A. *Mycoplasma*
0   B. *Neisseria meningitiditis*
0   C. Human immunodeficiency virus (HIV)
0   D. Epstein-Barr virus

Anaphylaxis

Mr. Barlage, a 34-year-old man, comes to the emergency department and states that he is having an allergic reaction to the seafood he just ate.

35. What presenting symptom would the emergency department nurse be most concerned with?
0   A. Urticaria
0   B. Wheezing
0   C. Anxiety
0   D. Nausea

36. The nursing diagnosis most appropriate for Mr. Barlage would be:
0   A. Knowledge deficit
0   B. Cardiac output, decreased
0   C. Gas exchange, impaired
0   D. Injury, potential for

37. The reaction will be treated with diphenhydramine, 25 mg IM. Prior to the administration of this medication, what question would be most appropriate for the emergency department nurse to ask?
0   A. "Are you planning on driving home?"
0   B. "How much do you weigh?"

0   C. "Are you allergic to anything?"

0   D. "Are you on any medication now?"

38. If the patient is allergic to seafood, there is a good chance that he may also be allergic to:

0   A. Iodine

0   B. Intravenous pyelogram (IVP) dye

0   C. Betadine

0   D. All of the above

39. Patient teaching on discharge should include which of the following?

0   A. Obtain a Medic-Alert tag

0   B. Always carry diphenhydramine

0   C. Avoid all forms of penicillin

0   D. Always carry epinephrine

Alcohol-Related Problems

40. Acute alcohol withdrawal and/or delirium tremens (DTs) occur during hospitalization primarily within these time frames:

0   A. During the first 12 hours

0   B. Within 72 hours

0   C. Within 5 to 7 days

0   D. They may occur at virtually any time

41. When obtaining a history from an alcoholic patient, the emergency nurse needs to remember that the patient's primary coping mechanism in responding to the questions will be:

0   A. Denial

0   B. Anger

0   C. Projection

0   D. Sublimation

42. Which of the following are the drugs of choice to prevent the onset of alcohol withdrawal?

0   A. Meperidine (Demerol) and promethazine (Phenergan)

0   B. Haloperidol (Haldol) and chlorpromazine (Thorazine)

0   C. Chlordiazepoxide (Librium) and diazepam (Valium)

0   D. Chlordiazepoxide (Librium) and disulfiram (Antabuse)

43. Patients with chronic alcoholism can have serious systemic effects from

their alcohol intake. What two common problems are seen in alcoholic patients in the emergency department?
  0 A. Confusion and urinary retention
  0 B. Lower gastrointestinal bleeding and epistaxis
  0 C. Dehydration and malnutrition
  0 D. Psychoses and pneumonia

44. A 28-year-old intoxicated man comes to the emergency department with an open fracture of his right tibia and fibula. His alcohol level is 189. He is oriented, and there is no evidence of head injury. His vital signs are blood pressure, 144/94; pulse, 104; and respiratory rate, 24. The physician orders meperidine (Demerol), 50 mg, and promethazine (Phenergan), 25 mg IM, stat for pain. The nurse should:
  0 A. Refuse to give the medication
  0 B. Give the medication and monitor the patient's vital signs
  0 C. Give the medication and have intubation equipment, a cardiac monitor, and a defibrillator ready
  0 D. Ask the patient if he really is in any pain

Diabetic Ketoacidosis

Ms. Gleason, a 25-year-old woman, is brought to the emergency department by her husband with a history of "the flu" of 3 day's duration. Ms. Gleason states that she has had nausea, vomiting and diarrhea, frequent urination, and a fever during this time. She has no medical history of diabetes. Her blood glucose level is 850.

45. Frequent factors that contribute to diabetic ketoacidosis (DKA) include all of the following *except:*
  0 A. Infection
  0 B. Water intoxication
  0 C. Stress
  0 D. Noncompliance

46. Ms. Gleason's breathing is rapid and deep, her respiratory rate is 38, and she has a fruity breath odor. This respiratory pattern is known as:
  0 A. Biot's respirations
  0 B. Cluster breathing
  0 C. Kussmaul's respirations
  0 D. Central neurogenic hyperventilation

47. Ms. Gleason's vital signs are blood pressure, 102/50; pulse, 120; respira-

tory rate, 38; and temperature, 101° F. Her potassium level is 2.8. What IV fluids should be given?

   0   A. Dextrose 5% with 0.45% NaCl with KCl, 20 mEq at 200 ml/hr

   0   B. 0.45% NaCl with KCl, 40 mEq at 200 ml/hr

   0   C. Ringer's lactate solution at wide-open rate

   0   D. Dextrose 5% in water (D_5W) at keep-open rate

48. The drug of choice to treat DKA with a glucose level of 800 is:

   0   A. Regular insulin

   0   B. Lente insulin

   0   C. Semilente insulin

   0   D. Glyburide (Micronase, Diabeta)

49. In treating Ms. Gleason, the emergency department personnel would want her blood glucose to be decreased to what level?

   0   A. 80 to 110

   0   B. Less than 200

   0   C. Less than 400

   0   D. Less than 500

Meningitis

50. The bacteria that causes meningitis can enter the meninges via:

   0   A. A basilar skull fracture

   0   B. Sinusitis

   0   C. A brain abscess

   0   D. All of the above

51. Bacterial meningitis and viral meningitis can be differentiated on a lumbar puncture by the following:

   0   A. A bacterial infection will have a low WBC count

   0   B. A bacterial infection will have a high WBC count

   0   C. A viral infection will have a high WBC count

   0   D. They cannot be differentiated by a lumbar puncture

52. Assessment findings in a patient with meningitis may include all of the following *except:*

   0   A. Kernig's sign

   0   B. An altered mental status

   0   C. Bradycardia

   0   D. Photophobia

53. An early indication of deterioration in a patient with meningitis would be:
0 A. Cushing's triad
0 B. A change or decrease in the level of consciousness
0 C. Status epilepticus
0 D. Fever and chills

54. Management of meningitis encompasses which of the following?
0 A. IV fluids for hydration and antibiotic therapy
0 B. Vital signs and neurological assessment
0 C. Seizure precautions
0 D. All of the above

Electrolyte Disorders

55. The most serious priority with hypokalemia is:
0 A. Cardiac dysrhythmias
0 B. Petit mal seizures
0 C. Muscle cramps
0 D. Vein irritation from IV KCl

56. A classic sign of hypocalcemia is:
0 A. Chvostek's sign
0 B. Grey Turner's sign
0 C. Homans' sign
0 D. Brudzinski's sign

57. A classic sign of severe hyponatremia is:
0 A. Cardiac arrest
0 B. Blurred vision
0 C. Seizures
0 D. A salty taste to the skin

58. In administering large volumes of Ringer's lactate solution to a patient in shock, the emergency department nurse should remember that:
0 A. Each 1000 ml contains 4.4 mEq of potassium
0 B. Each 1000 ml contains 40 mEq of potassium
0 C. There is no potassium in Ringer's lactate solution
0 D. Furosemide (Lasix) should be given to help rid the body of extra potassium

59. Patients with heat-related emergencies are prone to what problem?

0   A. Sudden-death dysrhythmias
0   B. Hypothalamus infarctions
0   C. Fluid retention
0   D. Fluid and electrolyte loss

Transplant Patients

60. An 18-year-old victim of multiple trauma is brought to the emergency department. He has massive head trauma with much gray matter visible. His right pupil is fixed and dilated, and he is completely nonresponsive, with a Glasgow Coma Scale rating of 3. His blood pressure is 80/60, and his pulse is 40; there is no respiratory effort. He is intubated, and his lungs are being manually ventilated. Nursing actions and goals should now be directed toward:

0   A. Suturing the head wounds and elevating the head of the bed 30 degrees
0   B. Maintaining perfusion and beginning to evaluate the potential for organ donation
0   C. Preparing the patient for the operating room
0   D. Treating hypovolemic shock

61. What would be a major barrier to any organ donation with the above patient?

0   A. The patient tests HIV positive
0   B. The patient was taking penicillin for an upper urinary tract infection prior to the accident
0   C. No driver's license permit for donations was signed
0   D. The potential for trauma to other organs

62. Mr. Borchers, who has been traveling on vacation, is brought to the emergency department of a small rural hospital (50 beds) by his wife. Six months earlier he had a heart transplant at a large university hospital that is several hours away. Now he is complaining of feeling short of breath. He is in atrial fibrillation with a rate of 120. His condition is serious but stable. An appropriate nursing action that would probably provide Mr. Borchers with the best care would be to:

0   A. Immediately tell Mrs. Borchers that the hospital is not equipped to handle this case and suggest that she drive her husband to the university hospital where he had his surgery.
0   B. Obtain immunological laboratory data as soon as possible.

0   C. Admit Mr. Borchers to the special care unit and treat him as any other stable cardiac patient.

0   D. Notify the transplant center at the university hospital of the patient's condition and ask them for guidelines for his care and/or possible transfer.

63. A common drug used for immunosuppression in transplant patients is:
0   A. Cyclosporine
0   B. Diphenhydramine (Benadryl)
0   C. Cryoprecipitate
0   D. Indomethacin (Indocin)

64. A chronic rejection usually occurs over a period of months to years. Regardless of the organ transplanted, which of the following patients may possibly be having a rejection?
0   A. Forty-four-year-old white man; WBC, 7500; hemoglobin, 13.2; blood pressure, 128/82; pulse, 84 (normal sinus rhythm); respiratory rate, 24
0   B. Sixty-year-old white man; WBC, 9000; respiratory rate, 36; audible rales; states "I can't get my breath!"
0   C. Thirty-nine-year-old black man; temperature, 99.9° F; complains of dizziness, pain, and weight gain; states "I just don't feel quite right."
0   D. Fifty-five-year-old white woman; blood pressure, 92/60; temperature, 104.4° F; WBC, 32,000; complains of "feeling hot all over"

ANSWERS

1. **B. Assessment.** Maintaining an airway is always the first priority. Determination of other injuries or problems will be done later through CT and arterial blood gas (ABG) assessment.

2. **C. Assessment/intervention.** Frequently coma may be due to hypoglycemia and/or drug overdose. Giving dextrose 50% and naloxone is standard initial treatment for coma patients. The other modalities may be done later.

3. **D. Assessment.** Biot's respirations, or cluster breathing, is usually reflective of severe cerebral edema with medullary involvement. Cheyne-Stokes respirations are "staircase" patterned breathing with periods of intermittent apnea. Central neurogenic hyperventilation is rapid, deep breathing seen in cerebral edema as well. Kussmaul's respirations are rapid, deep breathing

seen in diabetic ketoacidosis, in which the patient is usually unconscious.

4. **A. Assessment.** The Glasgow Coma Scale measures the functional state of the brain as a whole—especially assessing from full consciousness to coma. This includes eye movements, verbal response, and motor response.

5. **D. Intervention.** Without oxygen or glucose, the brain will die within minutes. The damage is increasingly irreversible with time. Although the other substances do assist with brain functioning, oxygen and glucose are the most crucial.

6. **C. Assessment.** Because of high levels of uric acid, patients with gout are also prone to developing renal calculi, especially in chronic gout. Hyperuricemia does not necessarily make a person more prone to a myocardial infarction, stroke, or sepsis.

7. **A. Analysis.** Arthritis can be an extremely painful condition, especially on arising. The other nursing diagnoses listed would not be appropriate.

8. **B. Evaluation.** NSAIDs should always be taken with food or milk. They can erode mucosal surfaces of the stomach and cause nausea, vomiting, and, in more severe cases, gastrointestinal bleeding.

9. **D. Assessment.** Crepitus and deformity are usually indicative of a fracture and/or dislocation. The other symptoms listed are associated with joint pain of chronic or inflammatory origin.

10. **D. Assessment.** Vomiting and other gastrointestinal symptoms are usually not associated with sickle cell crisis. Pain, weakness, and fever are commonly seen.

11. **B. Intervention.** Hydration is crucial in preventing sickling of cells and possible organ ischemia. This is usually accomplished with large amounts of IV fluids. Prevention of infection is important, but hydration is more of a priority. Transfusion therapy and patient teaching are not indicated at this time.

12. **D. Evaluation.** Because of its cellular level, the complications of sickle cell crisis are systemic and potentially fatal.

13. **A. Evaluation.** When sickling subsides, the patient will usually report less pain and the temperature will return to normal. The urine output and hemoglobin should not be affected. Since the patient may be slightly tachycardiac, relief of pain is a much more reliable factor.

14. **C. Assessment.** Because of the intense and chronic pain associated with the disease, patients with sickle cell disease are prone to developing patterns of addiction and dependency. Septic shock and DIC may only occasionally be seen. Paralysis is rare.

15. **D. Assessment.** Symptoms of dehydration include nausea, vomiting, dehydration, fatigue, muscle cramps, fever, and enophthalmos (deeply

sunken eyes). Exopthalmos (protrusion of the eyeball) is found in hyperthyroidism, endocrine disorders, and cranial, space-occupying lesions.

16. **B. Assessment.** Dehydration is evidenced by an elevated BUN. The hematocrit is usually elevated and the serum osmolality is greater than 310 mOsm in dehydration.

17. **A. Analysis.** The greatest concern is with the fluid volume deficit. Gas exchange, tissue integrity, and urinary elimination do not appear to be affected at this point.

18. **A. Evaluation.** Bilateral rales would indicate a fluid volume excess. A urine output of 30 ml/hr would indicate adequate renal perfusion and function. A decrease in hemoglobin is common in dehydrated patients after the initiation of IV fluids because of the previous hemoconcentration. The normal CVP is 5 to 15 cm H_2O.

19. **C. Intervention.** Decreasing the patient's IV fluids and giving oxygen would be the best initial approach. Furosemide would be contraindicated, since her dehydration was just previously corrected. Inserting a Swan-Ganz catheter may be done later if she does not respond to treatment. Monitoring of vital signs and an ECG are more assessment factors and do not actually intervene in pulmonary edema.

20. **D. Intervention.** As always, the first priorities are airway and ventilation. Most hemophiliac bleeding episodes are minor, and although they are potentially serious, they can usually be initially managed appropriately by a community hospital. Coagulation studies would be indicated later, as would the administration of cryoprecipitate.

21. **B. Assessment.** The severity of the disease is directly related to the activity level of factor VIII. While factor II, prothrombin, and fibrinogen are important for blood coagulation, they are not directly related to hemophilia.

22. **A. Evaluation.** After a wound has been sutured, the patient with hemophilia should be observed for 4 hours. Bleeding may be absent at first because the initial coagulation step of platelet plug formation is not affected by hemophilia. Cryoprecipitate is not indicated. Tetanus toxoid injections are given with care maintained to observe the injection site.

23. **A. Analysis.** The nursing diagnosis for Barry's mother is knowledge deficit. She is apparently unaware that acetylsalicylic acid (ASA) is contraindicated in hemophilia because of its anticoagulant properties. Also, joint pain may be a sign of occult bleeding in hemophiliac patients.

24. **B. Intervention.** IV fluids and cryoprecipitate are used to treat hemophiliac patients for hypovolemic shock. Vitamin K would not be appropriate.

25. **C. Assessment.** Congestive heart failure is rarely associated with a fever.

Appendicitis, meningitis, and PID are all infectious processes in which a fever is a predominant symptom.

26. **B. Intervention.** Pneumonia is a frequent cause of fever in the elderly. Therefore a chest x-ray film would be best to determine this problem. Testing for amylase and an ECG usually do not determine febrile conditions in the elderly, nor does a CT scan.

27. **A. Assessment.** Children are prone to febrile seizures. These result from how fast the temperature rises rather than how high. Epilepsy is defined as recurrent seizures and frequently occurs after head trauma. Meningitis is a cause of a seizure, rather than a result. Rarely do children arrest during or after a seizure, and if they do, it may be due to airway obstruction.

28. **D. Intervention.** Blankets would increase the core body temperature. A light sheet or one light blanket may be used. Cultures, IV fluids, antipyretics, and antibiotics are all indicated.

29. **B. Evaluation.** Children should not be given ASA because of the increased incidence of Reye's syndrome associated with ASA administration. The other statements reflect the parents' understanding of caring for a child with a fever.

30. **C. Assessment.** Orchiditis and fever can cause sterility in men. Gynecomastia and impotence are not associated with mumps. Oophoritis is inflammation of the ovaries (obviously found only in females).

31. **A. Assessment.** Pertussis is most commonly seen in children who have not been properly immunized. Many experts consider this to be a form of child neglect. *Haemophilus influenzae*, pollutants, and ASA misuse have no relationship to pertussis.

32. **A. Assessment.** Rubella is dangerous in the first trimester of pregnancy because it may cause fetal injuries that lead to deafness, mental retardation, cataracts, and birth defects.

33. **C. Assessment.** Chickenpox begins initially on the back and chest, and then progresses to the head and limbs. The perineal area may be involved in more severe cases.

34. **D. Assessment.** The Epstein-Barr virus is directly responsible for mononucleosis. *Mycoplasma* is a fungus that causes pneumonia. *Neisseria meningitiditis* is the causative agent for meningitis, and HIV is the virus that causes AIDS.

35. **B. Assessment.** Wheezing can indicate respiratory compromise, and airway maintenance is the first priority in an allergic reaction. Urticaria, anxiety, and nausea are less threatening indications of an allergic reaction.

36. **C. Analysis.** Wheezing can indicate impaired gas exchange. The other nursing diagnoses are not applicable at this time.

37. **A. Intervention.** Diphenhydramine causes drowsiness. Patients cannot drive after receiving this medication. In an adult, knowledge of weight is not crucial prior to the administration of this drug. Obviously, the patient is allergic to something, and the drug is indicated. Asking the patient if he is taking any medications should have been done on his arrival in the emergency department.

38. **D. Assessment.** Because seafood contains iodine, patients can and should be considered allergic to Betadine (povidone-iodine) and all drugs.

39. **A. Intervention.** The patient should be instructed to wear a Medic-Alert tag. This reaction was not very serious, so there is no need to carry drugs for injection yet. An allergy to seafood does not predispose the patient to be allergic to penicillin.

40. **D. Assessment.** Withdrawal and delirium symptoms from the cessation of alcohol may occur at any time during hospitalization. They may even occur when the blood alcohol level falls significantly below the patient's normal level.

41. **A. Assessment.** Practically everything that has to do with alcoholism centers around this denial. The patient, the family, and friends will use denial, and sometimes even physicians and nurses will. An alcoholic patient may project, become angry, or sublimate, but these behaviors are much less frequent than denial.

42. **C. Intervention.** Chlordiazepoxide is the drug of choice for the prevention of alcohol withdrawal symptoms. It is frequently used in conjunction with an antianxiety drug such as diazepam or lorazepam. Haloperidol may be used as well, but chlorpromazine is usually not needed. Several drugs in use today have eliminated the need for chlorpromazine. Disulfiram is used to prevent the alcoholic patient from consuming alcohol.

43. **C. Evaluation.** Because of the diuretic components of alcohol, practically all of these patients have some degree of dehydration. This is usually accompanied by malnutrition due to a decreased nutritional intake. Confusion and urinary retention are rare, as are psychosis and pneumonia. The bleeding that occurs in the gastrointestinal system is usually upper, not lower.

44. **B. Intervention.** Give the medication and monitor the patient's vital signs. The fracture that the patient has is painful and does warrant analgesic relief. The alcohol level, not the meperidine dose, is exceedingly high. If the nurse feels that after giving a medication, resuscitation equipment will be needed, it would be best not to give the drug at all. A patient with this type of fracture needs medication.

45. **B. Assessment.** Water intoxication does not contribute to the develop-

ment of DKA. Usually the patient is dehydrated and hypovolemic. Non-compliance is a major factor in DKA. Infection and stress may provoke this condition as well.

46. **C. Assessment.** Kussmaul's respirations are rapid, deep breathing frequently seen in DKA. The patient involuntarily breathes this way to correct the high CO_2 levels. Biot's respirations (also known as cluster breathing) and central neurogenic hyperventilation are indicative of increased intracranial pressure (ICP).

47. **B. Intervention.** Half-strength normal saline with KCl administered at a rapid rate is indicated to correct the patient's hypokalemia and hypo-volemia. No dextrose solutions should be used in DKA, because the glucose level is already elevated. Ringer's lactate solution may be indicated if her hypovolemia does not correct itself with the 0.45% NaCl.

48. **A. Intervention.** Regular insulin is the drug of choice because of its rapid, short-acting properties. Glyburide (Micronase, Diabeta) is an oral hypoglycemic agent for less serious cases of hyperglycemia. It would also be contraindicated because the patient is vomiting.

49. **B. Evaluation.** The goal would be to get the blood glucose level to lower than 200. If the blood glucose level gets too low (80 to 110), patients with previously or chronically high levels may develop hypoglycemic reactions.

50. **D. Assessment.** Bacteria can enter through all three of these routes. The three most common bacterial agents are *Streptococcus pneumoniae, Haemophilus influenzae,* and *Neisseria meningitidis.*

51. **B. Assessment.** On a lumbar puncture, a bacterial infection will be exhibited by a high WBC count (i.e., 2,000 to 20,000) with an elevated polymorphonuclear cell count. A viral infection will show a WBC count of less than 500.

52. **C. Assessment.** Bradycardia is a symptom generally not associated with meningitis. Kernig's sign (pain and resistance on extending the leg at the knee after flexing the thigh on the body), an altered mental status, and photophobia are all suggestive of meningeal irritation.

53. **B. Evaluation.** A change or decrease in the level of consciousness is an early sign of neurological deterioration and increased ICP. Cushing's triad comprises the three things (hypertension, pulse pressure widening, and bradycardia) seen later in severe increased ICP, as does status epilepticus. Fever and chills are early symptoms of meningitis, not neurological deterioration.

54. **D. Intervention.** The care of patients with meningitis includes all of these factors, with emphasis on detection and immediate intervention for complications.

55. **A. Assessment.** Cardiac dysrhythmias are a frequent and potentially dangerous complication of hypokalemia. Petit mal seizures may occur with hyponatremia. Muscle cramps (especially in the calf area) may occur with hypokalemia, as can vein irritation from IV KCl, but these are obviously less serious than dysrhythmias.

56. **A. Assessment.** Chvostek's sign, or facial twitching that occurs when the side of the face is tapped, is due to hypocalcemia. Grey Turner's sign, or ecchymosis of the flank area, is due to retroperitoneal bleeding. Homans' sign, or pain in the calf on dorsiflexion of the foot, is due to thrombophlebitis. Brudzinski's sign, or flexion of the hips and knees in response to flexion of the head and neck on the chest, is indicative of meningeal irritation.

57. **C. Assessment.** Grand mal seizures are very common in hyponatremia. Cardiac arrest can be seen in hypokalemia. Blurred vision is usually not found in hyponatremia. Children with cystic fibrosis have a salty taste to their skin.

58. **A. Intervention.** Each 1000 ml of Ringer's lactate solution contains about 4.4 mEq of potassium. Furosemide would be contraindicated in fluid resuscitation of shock unless severe overload were to occur.

59. **D. Assessment.** Most patients with heat exhaustion undergo fluid and electrolyte depletion. This loss can usually be corrected with Gatorade and/or IV fluids with concurrent cooling measures, depending on the severity of the problem. Sudden-death dysrhythmias may occur in severe hypokalemia or heat stroke. Infarction of the hypothalamus may occur secondary to a cerebrovascular accident (CVA).

60. **B. Intervention.** It is apparent that this injury is fatal. This patient would make an excellent candidate for organ donation. Efforts to maintain perfusion should be employed while concurrently advising the family about the potential outcome and making a request for donation. Suturing a head wound with gray matter visible would not be appropriate. Surgery, at this point, is not indicated. The patient is not in hypovolemic shock, because of the absence of tachycardia.

61. **A. Assessment.** Usually an HIV-positive finding is a serious threat to any potential organ donation. The fact that the patient was taking penicillin would be important but would not necessarily be a barrier to donation. Even if no driver's license consent has been signed, families may still donate organs. (Most patients who become organ donors have never signed a card.) There may be trauma to some organs, but others may be used.

62. **D. Intervention.** Patients receiving heart transplants are closely monitored for years after their surgery. Notification of the patient's physician

for stabilization and transfer is crucial. Mrs. Borchers should not drive the patient because of his condition and increased legal liability on the part of the rural hospital. The symptoms exhibited by Mr. Borchers seem to indicate congestive heart failure and not an allergic or rejection reaction. He needs a tertiary referral and probably should not be admitted to this hospital.

63. **A. Intervention.** Cyclosporine is an immunosuppressive agent used in transplantation. It is used in combination with azathioprine and prednisone. Diphenhydramine is an antihistamine. Cryoprecipitate is factor VIII used for hemophiliac patients. Indomethacin is a nonsteroidal anti-inflammatory drug.

64. **C. Assessment.** Not all possible signs and symptoms of rejection are present in every recipient or in every rejection episode. The patient may state that he or she "doesn't feel right." Dizziness, pain, weight gain, and fever may be the only symptoms present, but rejection may be occurring. Fever is a less common sign of rejection. Nurses should be on the alert for any subtle changes in the recipient's behavior and clinical status.

ADDITIONAL READINGS

Emergencies, Springhouse, PA, 1985, Springhouse.

Fincek M, Lanros N: *Emergency nursing: a comprehensive review,* Rockville, MD, 1986, Aspen.

Porth CM: *Pathophysiology,* ed 3, Philadelphia, 1990, JB Lippincott.

Rea R et al: *Emergency nursing core curriculum,* ed 3, Philadelphia, 1987, WB Saunders.

Rothberg MK: *Advanced medical life support: adult medical emergencies,* St Louis, 1987, Mosby–Year Book.

Chapter 7

Genitourinary and Gynecological Emergencies

REVIEW OUTLINE

I. Anatomy of the urinary tract
    A. Kidneys
    B. Ureter
    C. Bladder
    D. Urethra
    E. Renal vessels
    F. Urinary meatus
II. Anatomy of the male genital tract
    A. Seminal vesicles
    B. Prostate
    C. Corpus cavernosum
    D. Epididymis
    E. Testes
    F. Scrotum
    G. Spermatic cord
    H. Foreskin
    I. Glans penis
    J. Penile shaft
    K. Perineum
    L. Anus
III. Anatomy of the female genital tract
    A. Uterus
    B. Fallopian tubes
    C. Ovaries
    D. Cervix
    E. Vagina

F. Clitoris

G. Bartholin glands

H. Perineum

I. Anus

IV. Assessment and collaborative care of the patient with a genitourinary or gynecological emergency

   A. History

      1. Onset of problem (sudden or gradual)

      2. Last menstrual period

      3. Previous genitourinary and gynecological diseases or emergencies (e.g., previous ectopic pregnancy, sexually transmitted diseases)

      4. Urinary symptoms

         a. Dysuria

         b. Frequency

         c. Urgency

         d. Burning

         e. Hematuria

         f. Dribbling

         g. Incontinence

         h. Difficulty initiating urinary stream

      5. Gynecological symptoms

         a. Vaginal discharge (color, amount)

         b. Vaginal bleeding (color, amount, clots, or tissue)

         c. Vaginal itching

         d. Vaginal burning

      6. Medications

         a. Drugs that may interfere with urination

            (1) Antihistamines

            (2) Anticholinergics

            (3) Tricyclics

         b. Birth control devices

            (1) Birth control pills

            (2) Intrauterine device (IUD)

            (3) Diaphragm

         c. Hormones

      7. Medical problems

         a. Diabetes

         b. Renal disease

         c. Thyroid disorders

   B. Physical assessment

1. Location of pain
2. Associated signs and symptoms: nausea, vomiting, change in bowel functions
3. Fever, chills
4. Signs and symptoms of septic shock
5. External genitalia
6. Color of patient's urine
7. Amount of urine
8. Evaluation of hematuria
9. Auscultation of bowel sounds
10. Palpation and pelvic examination

C. Collaborative care
   1. Stabilization of ABCs (airway, breathing, circulation)
   2. Intravenous fluids
   3. Diagnostic studies or procedures
      a. Complete blood cell count (CBC) with differential
      b. Blood cultures when a fever is present
      c. Electrolytes, blood urea nitrogen (BUN), creatinine
      d. Beta human chorionic gonadotropin (BHCG; female patients of childbearing age)
      e. Urinalysis and urine culture
      f. Dipstick urine
      g. Ultrasound
      h. Intravenous pyelogram (IVP)

V. Related nursing diagnoses
   A. Anxiety
   B. Fluid volume deficit
   C. Hyperthermia (related to infection)
   D. Incontinence, urge
   E. Infection, potential for
   F. Knowledge deficit
   G. Pain (acute and chronic)
   H. Rape-trauma syndrome
   I. Urinary elimination, altered patterns
   J. Urinary retention

VI. Genitourinary and gynecological emergencies
   A. Renal trauma
   B. Bladder trauma
   C. Foreign bodies
   D. Kidney stone(s) (urolithiasis)

E. Urinary tract infection
F. Urinary retention
G. Hematuria
H. Renal failure
I. Torsion of the testicles
J. Epididymitis
K. Sexual assault
L. Vaginal bleeding
   1. Dysfunctional uterine bleeding
   2. Laceration
   3. Foreign bodies
   4. Sexual assault
M. Mittelschmerz
N. Ovarian cysts
O. Pelvic inflammatory disease
P. Sexually transmitted diseases
   1. Syphilis
   2. Gonorrhea
   3. Chlamydia
   4. Herpes simplex
   5. Condyloma acuminatum (venereal warts)
   6. Chancroid
   7. Granuloma inguinale
   8. Lymphogranuloma venereum

INTRODUCTION

*T*he assessment and care of the patient who is suffering from either a genitourinary or a gynecological emergency are based on obtaining a history of the chief complaint and then performing an evaluation of the patient's back, abdomen, urine, external genitalia, and pelvis. The assessment of the patient's complaint of urinary tract symptoms includes questioning the patient about dysuria, frequency, urgency, and hematuria. In addition, the emergency nurse should obtain a history of any vaginal, penile, or rectal discharge, including color, amount, odor, when it occurs, and how long it lasts.

For the female patient, assessment should include documentation of the patient's last menstrual period. The patient should be questioned about any problems with or differences in her period. Other factors to be considered when obtaining a menstrual history include the patient's age when her period began, the interval between her periods, the duration of the period, and the date of her last period.[1] If the patient is having vaginal bleeding or is complaining of a vaginal discharge, the emergency nurse needs to question the patient about the color and amount of the discharge, as well as the presence of clots or tissues.

The care of the patient with a genitourinary or gynecological emergency may include diagnostic studies: CBC, electrolytes, BUN, creatinine, BHCG for female patients of childbearing age, urinalysis, urinary culture, ultrasound, and IVP. Some gynecological and genitourinary emergencies cause the patient a great deal of pain. Pain management may include oral, intramuscular, or intravenous administration of medications, as well as providing the patient with comfort measures such as a warm blanket or a place to lie down.

The care of the patient who has been sexually assaulted can be very challenging for the emergency nurse. The patient who has suffered a sexual assault will require both physical and emotional care. In addition, because a crime has occurred, the emergency nurse is responsible for the collection and preservation of evidence.

The emergency nursing care of the patient with a genitourinary or gynecological emergency will depend on the origin of the emergency and the patient's response to it.

REVIEW QUESTIONS
Kidney Stone

A 48-year-old man comes to the emergency department complaining of abdominal pain and an inability to void. He states that he has been drinking a lot of water, taking acetaminophen (Tylenol) for pain, and using a heating pad on his abdomen.

1. The initial assessment of this patient should include:
   - 0 A. Palpation of peripheral pulses
   - 0 B. Determining the pattern of the patient's pain
   - 0 C. Discovering what type of diet the patient is on
   - 0 D. Obtaining a BUN and creatinine

2. The most common cause of kidney stones is:
   - 0 A. Oxalate
   - 0 B. Magnesium ammonium
   - 0 C. Uric acid
   - 0 D. Calcium oxalate

3. All of the following could contribute to this patient's inability to void *except:*
   0   A. Ingestion of eight glasses of water
   0   B. Taking 50 mg of amitriptyline (Elavil)
   0   C. Blunt trauma to the bladder
   0   D. Presence of a foreign body in the urethra

4. The patient is unable to void, and the emergency nurse will need to obtain a specimen through catheterization. What can the nurse do to make the procedure more comfortable?
   0   A. Give the patient some ice water to drink
   0   B. Tell the patient to take slow, deep breaths as the catheter is inserted
   0   C. Obtain an order to use lidocaine (Xylocaine) jelly to lubricate the catheter
   0   D. Consult a urologist to place the catheter because the patient has possible obstruction

5. The patient's IVP reveals a kidney stone, and the patient will be discharged home to pass the stone. The patient will be given oxycodone (Percodan) for pain and a strainer to use while voiding. An appropriate nursing diagnosis for the patient's home-going instructions would be:
   0   A. Fluid volume deficit related to renal calculi
   0   B. Pain related to penile discharge
   0   C. Urinary elimination, altered patterns, related to obstruction from a kidney stone
   0   D. Incontinence, urge, related to renal calculi

6. Audit criteria for the chart of this patient (or any patient who has been treated in the emergency department for renal calculi) should include documentation of:
   0   A. Hemoptysis
   0   B. Urinalysis
   0   C. Hematochezia
   0   D. A CBC with differential

Testicular Torsion

An 11-year-old boy is brought to the emergency department by his parents. They state that he had been climbing a tree and began suffering severe pain in his groin. The child is alert, diaphoretic, and obviously very uncomfortable.

7. It is important for the emergency nurse to include the following in the initial assessment of this child:
   0   A. History of urinary tract symptoms
   0   B. Psychosocial history
   0   C. History of hematochezia
   0   D. Immunization history

8. The diagnosis of testicular torsion has been made by the urologist. Manual manipulation of the testicle has failed to reduce the torsion. The emergency nurse will now prepare the patient and his family for:
   0   A. Care of the torsion at home
   0   B. Admission to the hospital for observation
   0   C. A barium enema to reduce the torsion
   0   D. Surgery for reduction of the torsion

9. The child becomes very upset when he is told that he must go to surgery for repair of the problem with his testicle. He becomes combative and states he will not go. The emergency nurse will plan the care of the patient using the following nursing diagnosis:
   0   A. Growth and development, altered, related to surgery
   0   B. Fear related to a potentially threatening situation
   0   C. Sexual dysfunction (potential for) related to testicular torsion
   0   D. Mobility, impaired physical

10. The emergency nurse provides the patient and his family with a private place in which to prepare for the surgery and spends time explaining the activities related to the surgery. The emergency nurse might observe which of the following if this intervention is effective?
   0   A. The patient's pulse rate increases to 150 when the nurse enters the room
   0   B. The patient turns his back when the nurse enters the room
   0   C. The patient verbalizes his fear of the surgery
   0   D. The patient's family takes the child home

Sexually Transmitted Diseases

11. A 22-year-old man comes to the emergency department complaining of scrotal swelling and pain. Epididymitis is diagnosed by the emergency medicine physician.

   The organism that frequently causes epididymitis in sexually active males is:

0 A. *Neisseria gonorrhoeae*
0 B. *Chlamydia trachomatis*
0 C. *Treponema pallidum*
0 D. *Escherichia coli*

12. A 20-year-old woman comes to the emergency department complaining of a rash on the palms of her hands and the soles of her feet. She states that it does not itch. The patient states that one of her sexual partners had been treated for a sexually transmitted disease 3 months earlier, but only recently told her. What sexually transmitted disease may be causing this rash?
0 A. Nongonococcal urethritis
0 B. Syphilis
0 C. Gonorrhoea
0 D. Herpes simplex II

13. Because some gonorrhea has been found to be penicillin resistant, the following drug has been recommended by the Centers for Disease Control for the treatment of gonorrhea:
0 A. Parenteral penicillin G
0 B. IV tetracycline
0 C. Ceftriaxone sodium
0 D. Aqueous penicillin

14. An appropriate nursing diagnosis for the patient who is being treated for a sexually transmitted disease in the emergency department would be:
0 A. Infection related to *Chlamydia trachomatis*
0 B. Knowledge deficit related to the etiology and treatment of pelvic inflammatory disease
0 C. Sexual dysfunction (potential for) related to the diagnosis of gonorrhea
0 D. Violence, potential for, related to the diagnosis of a sexually transmitted disease

15. A patient diagnosed as having a sexually transmitted disease is treated with an IM antibiotic. To evaluate the patient for the potential of an anaphylactic reaction to the medication, the emergency nurse should observe the patient for:
0 A. 24 hours
0 B. 30 minutes

0   C. 5 minutes

0   D. No observation is needed

Genitourinary Trauma

An 18-year-old man is brought to the emergency department after having been struck by a car while riding his bicycle. The patient was wearing a helmet. He is alert and oriented, complaining of back and abdominal pain. His vital signs are blood pressure, 80/40; pulse, 140; and respiratory rate, 28.

16. All of the following could indicate genitourinary trauma *except:*

0   A.   Coopernail's sign

0   B.   Costovertebral tenderness

0   C.   Grey Turner's sign

0   D.   Positive Homans' sign

17. A Foley catheter needs to be inserted in order for a peritoneal lavage to be performed. Which of the following would be a contraindication to insertion of the catheter?

0   A.   The patient has a pelvic fracture

0   B.   The patient complains of lower abdominal pain

0   C.   The patient is unconscious

0   D.   There is blood around the urinary meatus

18. The initial care of this patient would be based on the following nursing diagnosis:

0   A.   Injury, potential for, related to blunt force to the flank

0   B.   Infection, potential for, related to insertion of the catheter

0   C.   Fluid volume deficit related to hemorrhage

0   D.   Anxiety related to potential sexual dysfunction

19. Audit criteria for the chart of this patient (or any patient who has suffered genitourinary trauma) should include documentation of:

0   A.   Presence or absence of hematuria

0   B.   Presence of family in the emergency department

0   C.   Neurological assessment

0   D.   History of a sexually transmitted disease

Sexual Assault

A 30-year-old woman is brought to the emergency department by the police. The patient states that she was sexually assaulted on her way to work. The incident occurred about 2 hours earlier.

20. The initial assessment of the victim of sexual assault should include:
    0   A. Identification of any physical injuries the patient may have suffered
    0   B. The patient's emotional response to the sexual assault
    0   C. Who has accompanied the patient to the emergency department
    0   D. The amount of time it took the woman to report the assault

21. Clothing collected as evidence from the victim of a sexual assault should be:
    0   A. Labeled and left outside the patient's room
    0   B. Labeled and placed in a plastic bag
    0   C. Given back to the patient
    0   D. Labeled and placed in a paper bag

22. The nursing diagnosis on which the emergency nurse will base the care of this patient is:
    0   A. Posttrauma response
    0   B. Social isolation
    0   C. Rape-trauma syndrome
    0   D. Powerlessness

23. A short-term goal on which the emergency nurse could evaluate the care of this patient (or any victim of sexual assault) would be:
    0   A. The patient will return to her prior level of functioning
    0   B. The patient will leave the area
    0   C. The patient will have her physical needs met
    0   D. The patient will have support from her family while in the emergency department

Pyelonephritis

A 23-year-old woman comes to the emergency department complaining of a fever, chills, dysuria, and pain all over. The patient states that she has never had a kidney or bladder infection.

Based on the patient's urinalysis and CBC, the emergency medicine physician makes the diagnosis of acute pyelonephritis.

24. A common physical finding in the patient with pyelonephritis is:
    0   A. Tenderness over the affected flank area
    0   B. Tenderness behind both calves
    0   C. Tenderness in the upper extremities
    0   D. Tenderness over the sinuses

25. The patient is to be discharged from the emergency department. Discharge teaching for the patient diagnosed with acute pyelonephritis should include all of the following *except:*

   0   A.   Rest in bed as much as possible

   0   B.   Increase fluid intake to 3500 to 4000 ml per day

   0   C.   Only take the antibiotics until feeling better

   0   D.   Return if the pain increases

ANSWERS

1. **B. Assessment.** Determination of the location and pattern of the patient's pain will help the emergency nurse discover what the patient's problem is. The complaint of inability to void would have already alerted the emergency nurse to the possibility of a kidney stone. The location and pattern of the pain contributes additional information. The pain may be in different places depending on the location of the stone. Classic pain patterns for renal stones include pain in the flank area radiating to the groin, pain in the lower quadrant, and low back pain.[2]

2. **D. Assessment.** Seventy-five percent of renal stones result from calcium oxalate.[3]

3. **A. Assessment.** All of the answers except ingestion of fluids could contribute to the patient's inability to void. It is important for the emergency nurse to get a detailed history from the patient in relation to any potential problem that could cause the patient to be unable to void. Drugs such as antihistamines, anticholinergics, and antidepressants can cause urinary retention. Bladder trauma and the presence of a foreign body in the urethra could also interfere with the patient's ability to void.[2]

4. **C. Intervention.** Using copious amounts of lubricant—lidocaine jelly—can be helpful in making the procedure more comfortable for the patient. If the catheter will not pass, the obstruction site should be noted and the physician or urologist notified to prevent trauma to the urethra.[2]

5. **C. Analysis.** The patient will need to be taught about the use of the strainer while voiding and the use of pain medication and its effect on urinary elimination. The defining characteristics of this nursing diagnosis are dysuria, frequency, urinary retention, and change in amount, color, or odor of the urine.[4]

6. **B. Evaluation.** A urinalysis should be obtained on all patients with complaints of urinary symptoms. The color, amount, odor, and presence or absence of blood should be documented on the chart.

7. **A. Assessment.** To confirm the possibility of testicular torsion, which is a very serious emergency, the emergency nurse needs to gather data about what other problems the patient could be experiencing, with related signs and symptoms. Even though the patient's onset of symptoms indicate the possibility of torsion, urinary tract infections and muscle pulls can also cause severe pain.[5]

8. **D. Intervention.** To ensure testicular salvage, the torsion needs to be reduced within 6 hours. If manual manipulation is attempted and fails, the patient will need to have surgery performed for detorsion of the testes.[2]

9. **B. Analysis.** The emergency nursing care of this patient would be planned using the nursing diagnosis of fear related to a potentially life-threatening situation, which would be the surgery. The defining characteristics of this nursing diagnosis include terror, fight behavior, flight behavior, and panic.[4]

10. **C. Evaluation.** The patient's ability to verbalize his fears about the surgery would help the emergency nurse evaluate the effectiveness of the interventions.[4]

11. **B. Assessment.** The most common organism causing epididymitis in a sexually active male patient is *Chlamydia trachomatis*. It may account for over two thirds of the cases of epididymitis.[2]

12. **B. Assessment.** The clinical manifestations of secondary syphilis include mucocutaneous lesions that occur in 80% of patients with the disease. The mucotaneous lesions appear on the palate, pharynx, glans of the penis, and vulva. The rashes that occur in secondary syphilis do not itch and can be macular, papular, pustular, or squamous lesions. They frequently appear bilaterally on the palms of the hands or soles of the patient's feet.[5,6]

13. **C. Intervention.** Ceftriaxone sodium has been recommended for the treatment of penicillin-resistant gonorrhea. This drug can still be painful when administered. To decrease the pain, it can be reconstituted with lidocaine.[1]

14. **B. Analysis.** The most important and valuable care that the emergency nurse can provide for the patient being treated for a sexually transmitted disease in the emergency department is to provide the patient with information about the disease process and the appropriate treatment regimen that the patient should follow to prevent the problems that could result.

15. **B. Evaluation.** After the patient has been given an IM antibiotic, the patient should be instructed to remain in the emergency department area

for 30 minutes so that if any complications should occur, the patient can be quickly treated.[7]

16. **D. Assessment.** The emergency nurse should suspect the possibility of genitourinary trauma with the presence of Coopernail's sign (ecchymosis of the labia or scrotum), Grey Turner's sign (ecchymosis of the flank area), and costovertebral tenderness (fractures of the lower ribs and the vertebrae).[3]

17. **D. Intervention.** Blood at the urinary meatus is an indication of an injury to the urethra. Before the catheter is passed, a urethrogram should be obtained.[2,5]

18. **A. Analysis.** Based on the patient's vital signs on arrival in the emergency department, the initial care of this patient would be directed at correcting hemorrhagic shock.

19. **A. Evaluation.** The presence or absence of hematuria should be documented for all patients who have suffered genitourinary trauma.

20. **A. Assessment.** The initial assessment of any victim of a violent crime should be focused on identification of any physical injuries that could potentially be life threatening.[5,7]

21. **D. Intervention.** All evidence that is collected needs to be labeled with the patient's name, date, time of collection, and who collected the evidence. Evidence such as clothing should be placed in a clean paper bag. Paper bags should be used instead of plastic so that moisture does not collect and destroy the evidence.[8]

22. **C. Analysis.** Unfortunately, the occurrence of sexual assault remains one of our society's major social ills. Nursing interacts with the victims of sexual assault not only in the emergency department, but within the hospital and the community as well. Because of the complex care required by these victims (males, females, children, young and old adults), specific nursing diagnoses have been developed. These include rape-trauma syndrome; rape-trauma syndrome: silent reaction; and rape-trauma syndrome: compound reaction.[4]

23. **C. Evaluation.** An obtainable short-term goal for the emergency department nurse would be meeting the physical needs of the victim of sexual assault. Although the patient is going to need follow-up and support from family and friends, these are long-term goals that may not be met during the emergency department visit.[7]

24. **A. Assessment.** Signs and symptoms of pyelonephritis include chills, fever, urinary urgency and frequency, and tenderness over the affected flank area.[5]

25. **C. Intervention.** The patient should be instructed to take all of the antibiotics prescribed.

REFERENCES

1. Stine R, Marcus R: *A practical approach to emergency medicine,* Boston, 1987, Little, Brown.
2. Keeler T, Carter: Genitourinary emergencies. In Kitt S, Kaiser J, editors: *Emergency nursing: a physiologic and clinical perspective,* Philadelphia, 1990, WB Saunders.
3. Thomas HA, O'Conner R, Hoffman G: *Emergency medicine: self-assessment and review,* ed 2, St Louis, 1988, Mosby–Year Book.
4. McFarland GK, McFarlane EA: *Nursing diagnosis and intervention: planning for patient care,* St Louis, 1989, Mosby–Year Book.
5. Sheehy SB: *Mosby's manual of emergency care,* ed 3, St Louis, 1990, Mosby–Year Book.
6. Levine J: Syphilis: ancient and on the rise, *Emerg Med* 5:62-73, 1988.
7. Reedy N, Brucker M: Obstetric and gynecologic emergencies. In Kitt S, Kaiser J, editors: *Emergency nursing: a physiologic and clinical perspective,* Philadelphia, 1990, WB Saunders.
8. Sexual assault protocol, University of Cincinnati Hospital, Cincinnati, 1990.

Chapter 8

Neurological Emergencies

REVIEW OUTLINE
I. Anatomy and physiology
   A. Anatomy
      1. Scalp
      2. Skull
      3. Meninges
         a. Dura mater
         b. Arachnoid
         c. Pia mater
      4. Brain
         a. Cerebrum
         b. Cerebellum
         c. Brainstem
   B. Physiology
      1. Neurons
      2. Neurotransmitters
      3. Central nervous system
         a. Frontal lobe
         b. Parietal lobe
         c. Occipital lobe
         d. Temporal lobe
      4. Limbic lobe
      5. Basal ganglia
      6. Pons
      7. Medulla oblongata
      8. Reticular activating system
      9. Spinal cord
         a. Ascending pathways
         b. Descending pathways

10. Peripheral nervous system
    a. Cranial nerves
    b. Spinal nerves
11. Autonomic nervous system
    a. Sympathetic
    b. Parasympathetic
12. Circle of Willis
13. Cerebrospinal fluid
C. Intracranial pressure (ICP)
    1. ICP = volume of brain tissue + volume of blood + volume of cerebrospinal fluid
    2. Cerebral perfusion pressure = mean arterial blood pressure − mean intracranial pressure
D. Nutrients of the brain and spinal cord
    1. Glucose
    2. Oxygen

II. Neurological assessment
    A. Level of consciousness
    B. Pupillary response
    C. Motor response
    D. Sensory response
    E. Vital signs
    F. History

III. Collaborative care of the patient with a neurological emergency
    A. Airway: neurogenic influences, seizure activity, oxygen
    B. Breathing: hyperventilation
    C. Circulation: hypotension
    D. Neurological deficit: baseline neurological assessment
    E. Immobilization of the cervical spine
    F. History of illness or injury, past medical history, current medications
    G. Control of ICP
        1. Recognition of the signs and symptoms of increasing ICP
        2. Elevation of the bed, decreased stimulation
        3. Airway stabilization with hyperventilation; monitoring of blood gases when hyperventilation is being used
        4. Medications
            a. Mannitol
            b. Furosemide (Lasix)
            c. Phenobarbital
            d. Phenytoin (Dilantin)
            e. Others

H. Laboratory tests
1. Drug screen
2. ETOH (blood alcohol level)
3. Hemoglobin and hematocrit
4. Lumbar puncture
I. Radiography
1. Cervical spine elevation
2. Computed tomography (CT) scan
3. Magnetic resonance imaging (MRI)
J. Cervical traction
K. ICP monitoring
IV. Related nursing diagnoses
A. Airway clearance, ineffective
B. Anxiety
C. Breathing pattern, ineffective
D. Fear
E. Gas exchange, impaired
F. Grieving, anticipatory
G. Home maintenance management, impaired
H. Hopelessness
I. Infection, potential for
J. Injury, potential for
K. Knowledge deficit
L. Pain
M. Powerlessness
N. Spiritual distress (distress of the human spirit)
O. Swallowing, impaired
P. Tissue perfusion, altered (cerebral or spinal cord)
V. Specific neurological emergencies
A. Headache
B. Cerebrovascular accident (CVA)
C. Seizures
D. Coma
E. Infections
F. Subarachnoid bleeding, aneurysms
G. Bell's palsy
H. Skull fractures
1. Periorbital ecchymosis
2. Cerebrospinal fluid leaking
3. Battle's sign
4. Palpable depression

I.   Concussion
J.   Mild head injuries
   1. Coma scale: 13 to 15
   2. No focal neurological signs or symptoms
   3. Negative findings on the CT scan
K. Moderate head injury
   1. Coma scale: 9 to 12
   2. Focal neurological findings
   3. Positive findings on the CT scan
   4. Requires interventions
L.   Severe head injuries
   1. Coma scale: 8 or less
   2. Neurological findings
   3. Injury noted on the CT scan
   4. Requires interventions
M. Contusion
N. Bleeds
   1. Subdural hematoma
   2. Epidural hematoma
   3. Intracerebral hematoma
O. Surface trauma
   1. Scalp lacerations
   2. Facial abrasions
P.   Low back pain
Q. Spinal cord injuries
   1. History
   2. Neurological assessment
   3. Radiographic evaluation
   4. Level of the injury
   5. Spinal shock

INTRODUCTION

*T*he care of the patient who is suffering from a neurological emergency can be very challenging to the emergency nurse. Neurological emergencies are classified as having a medical or surgical origin, even though some of these emergencies may be treated both medically and surgically.

One of the most frequent neurological emergencies encountered by the emergency nurse is head trauma. About 500,000 head injuries occur annually, and about one half of these reach the hospital.[1] Head trauma is the most common injury that occurs in the pediatric population.[2]

The initial stabilization and management of the patient who has suffered a neurological emergency is based on several factors, including continuous neurological assessment, immobilization of the cervical spine (when trauma is suspected), and management of increased intracranial pressure (ICP). It is important to review the mechanism of increased ICP, as well as its management. Some of the references listed at the end of the chapter may be of help.

The emergency nurse should always immobilize the cervical spine of any patient who is suspected of sustaining a head injury. The Trauma Nurse Core Curriculum (TNCC) provides in-depth information about cervical spine immobilization.

A baseline neurological assessment consists of five components: level of consciousness (Glasgow Coma Scale, Modified Glasgow Coma Scale, AVPU method [alert, response to verbal and painful stimuli, unresponsiveness]); pupillary response; motor response; sensory response; and vital signs. Other information that can provide additional clues to the patient's neurological status include the patient's past medical history, history related to the present illness or injury, and current medications.

REVIEW QUESTIONS
Seizures

A 50-year-old man is brought to the emergency department by ground ambulance. He has multiple abrasions on his face. On arrival in the emergency department, the patient is having a generalized seizure and is cyanotic. An IV line has been established.

1. What drug should be administered first to control this patient's seizures?
   0   A. Phenytoin sodium
   0   B. Diazepam
   0   C. Phenobarbital sodium
   0   D. Fentanyl

2. This patient has a documented history of seizures and alcohol abuse. What other pieces of history should be obtained about this patient during the initial assessment?
   0   A. Any recent falls or blows to the head
   0   B. Medication compliance
   0   C. The amount of alcohol he has ingested
   0   D. His family physician

3. The patient begins having another seizure. What is the primary nursing diagnosis on which the emergency nurse should base care?
   0   A. Swallowing, impaired
   0   B. Thought processes, altered
   0   C. Airway clearance ineffective
   0   D. Injury, potential for

4. The emergency medicine physician has ordered that the patient be given 500 mg of phenytoin intravenously. The patient is placed on a cardiac monitor, and the infusion is started. What criterion should the emergency nurse use to evaluate the toxic effects of the drug?
   0   A. No noted seizure activity
   0   B. Bradycardia
   0   C. Nausea and vomiting
   0   D. Sinus rhythm

Febrile seizures

An 18-month-old boy is brought to the emergency department by his parents, who say that the child has been "shaking" and clenching his teeth for about 15 minutes. They also state that he has not been feeling well for the past 2 days.

5. All of the following would suggest that the child is suffering from a febrile seizure *except* a:
   0   A. Family history of seizures
   0   B. Recent upper respiratory tract infection
   0   C. Fall from his crib
   0   D. Recent immunization

6. Because of his generalized seizure activity, an IV line cannot be established. What other route would ensure a rapid response to the anticonvulsant?
   0   A. Oral
   0   B. Intramuscular
   0   C. Subcutaneous
   0   D. Intraosseous

7. During the child's seizure activity, the emergency nurse observes that the child's lips are cyanotic. What is the most appropriate nursing diagnosis on which the emergency nurse could base care?
   0   A. Injury, potential for
   0   B. Thought processes, altered

0   C. Gas exchange, impaired
0   D. Growth and development, altered

8. Phenobarbital has been prescribed for the child by the emergency physician. What should the parents be taught about the side effects of this drug?
0   A. The drug will initially cause drowsiness
0   B. The drug may cause mental retardation
0   C. The drug may cause overgrowth of the child's gums
0   D. The drug may discolor the child's teeth

Headache and Cerebrovascular Accident

A 24-year-old woman comes to the emergency department complaining of severe pain in her head. She states no history of any medical problems.

9. Common signs and symptoms associated with migraine headaches include:
0   A. Unilateral pupillary changes
0   B. Grand mal seizures
0   C. Photophobia, nausea, and vomiting
0   D. Ventricular fibrillation

10. For any patient with the complaint of headache, in addition to an evaluation of the ABCs (airway, breathing, circulation), the following assessment should be performed:
0   A. Level of consciousness
0   B. Palpation of peripheral pulses
0   C. Deep tendon reflexes
0   D. Abdominal assessment

11. A drug that has been found to be effective in the acute management of migraine headache is:
0   A. Meperidine intravenously
0   B. Acetaminophen rectally
0   C. Naproxen orally
0   D. Dihydroergotamine (DHE) intravenously

12. Other emergency nursing interventions that will help relieve the pain of a headache include:
0   A. Application of a hot pack to the patient's forehead
0   B. Application of a cold cloth to the patient's forehead

    0   C. Having the patient sit in the waiting room after medication
administration

    0   D. Leaving the lights on in the examining room

13. A relevant nursing diagnosis for the emergency nursing care of the
patient with a headache would be:
    0   A. Social isolation
    0   B. Tissue integrity, impaired
    0   C. Pain (acute)
    0   D. Knowledge deficit

14. The emergency physician has ordered that the patient be given IV
prochlorperazine for her nausea. Before discharge, the patient should be
evaluated for:
    0   A. Changes in pupillary function
    0   B. Orthostatic hypotension
    0   C. The presence of a rash
    0   D. Diaphoresis

*An 80-year-old man has been brought to the emergency department by his family.
They state that he has been walking "funny," they cannot understand what he says,
the left side of his face is drooping, and he is not using his left arm.*

15. The emergency nurse performs a cranial nerve assessment on the
patient during the initial neurological evaluation. Which cranial
nerves control the motor and sensory function of the patient's facial
movement?
    0   A. I and II (olfactory and optic)
    0   B. IV and V (trochlear and trigeminal)
    0   C. X and XI (vagus and spinal accessory)
    0   D. V and VII (trigeminal and facial)

16. A heparin drip has been ordered to treat the patient's diagnosed
thrombotic stroke. Heparin (10,000 units) is added to 500 ml of
dextrose 5% in water (D_5W). It is to run at 1000 units per hour.
How many milliliters per hour should the IV monitor be set at?
(The IV set delivers 10 gtt/ml.)
    0   A. 25 ml/hr
    0   B. 20 ml/hr
    0   C. 100 ml/hr
    0   D. 5 ml/hr

17. From the data collected during the nursing assessment of this patient, his plan of care in the emergency department should be based on which of the following nursing diagnoses?
    - 0   A. Tissue perfusion, altered (cerebral)
    - 0   B. Social isolation
    - 0   C. Skin integrity, impaired, potential
    - 0   D. Mobility, impaired physical

18. During the administration of heparin, the emergency nurse should evaluate the patient for:
    - 0   A. Cardiac dysrhythmia
    - 0   B. Acute bleeding
    - 0   C. Peripheral edema
    - 0   D. Abdominal distention

Infection

A 3-year-old boy is brought to the emergency department by his parents. They state that he has been lethargic, febrile, and vomiting. He was recently treated for an inner ear infection. The patient's vital signs are blood pressure, 70/40; pulse, 160; respiratory rate, 40; and temperature (rectal), 103° F.

19. During the initial evaluation of this child, the emergency nurse should also assess for:
    - 0   A. Positive Kernig's or Brudzinski's signs
    - 0   B. Occulocephalic reflex
    - 0   C. Deep tendon reflexes
    - 0   D. Romberg test

20. Based on the patient's history and physical examination, the *initial* care of this patient should be:
    - 0   A. A lumbar puncture
    - 0   B. Administration of antibiotics
    - 0   C. Stabilization of his shock
    - 0   D. Obtaining a CT scan

21. A set of arterial blood gases is obtained. The results are pH, 7.15; Po_2, 60; Pco_2, 20; and HCO_3, 18. These blood gases indicate:
    - 0   A. Respiratory alkalosis
    - 0   B. Metabolic acidosis
    - 0   C. Respiratory acidosis
    - 0   D. Metabolic alkalosis

22. The child's presenting blood pressure and pulse indicate that the emergency nurse should base the initial care on which of the following nursing diagnoses?
    0   A. Thermoregulation, ineffective
    0   B. Fluid volume deficit
    0   C. Fluid volume, excess
    0   D. Tissue integrity, impaired

23. A Foley catheter is inserted. What criteria should the emergency nurse use to evaluate adequate urinary output during the fluid resuscitation?
    0   A. Urine output greater than 1 ml/kg/hr
    0   B. Urine output less than 1 ml/kg/hr
    0   C. Urine output less than 0.5 ml/kg/hr
    0   D. Urine output greater than 0.5 ml/kg/hr

Head and Spinal Trauma

An 18-year-old man is brought by helicopter to the emergency department after a motorcycle accident. At the scene of the accident, the patient was awake but combative. His initial Glasgow Coma Scale rating was 12. On his arrival in the emergency department, the patient's Glasgow Coma Scale rating is 7. He has abrasions on his face, and both eyes are ecchymotic and swollen shut.

24. The presence of periorbital ecchymosis in a patient with an altered mental status may indicate a:
    0   A. Maxillary fracture
    0   B. Basilar skull fracture
    0   C. Hemothorax
    0   D. Nasal fracture

25. An additional indication of a skull fracture would be:
    0   A. A hemotympanic membrane
    0   B. A fracture of the first rib
    0   C. An eyebrow laceration
    0   D. Hyperhidrosis

26. Because of the possibility of a skull fracture, the emergency nurse should avoid:
    0   A. Placing a cervical collar on the patient
    0   B. Placing an oral airway in the patient
    0   C. Inserting a nasogastric tube
    0   D. Placing the patient on a cardiac monitor

27. The patient is orally intubated by the emergency physician. He is being hyperventilated, but his neurological condition does not improve. His pupils are now 6 mm bilaterally and slow to react. His Glasgow Coma Scale rating has decreased to 5. The emergency physician orders mannitol to be infused. The patient weighs 100 kg. How much mannitol will be initially infused?

  0   A. 100 g
  0   B. 50 g
  0   C. 500 g
  0   D. 25 g

28. Intracranial pressure is the result of:

  0   A. The volume of brain tissue plus the volume of blood plus the volume of cerebrospinal fluid
  0   B. The mean arterial blood pressure minus the mean intracranial pressure
  0   C. O_2 plus a glucose level above 100
  0   D. An increase in the mean arterial pressure

29. The patient begins having copious amounts of pink, frothy sputum coming from his endotracheal tube. The emergency nurse should base the care for this complication on which of the following nursing diagnoses?

  0   A. Cardiac output, decreased
  0   B. Gas exchange, impaired
  0   C. Hypothermia
  0   D. Fluid volume deficit

A 2-year-old boy has been brought to the emergency department by the EMTs. He was involved in a motor vehicle crash with his parents, and at the time was restrained on his mother's lap by a shoulder harness. On arrival of the EMTs, the child was in full cardiac arrest. CPR was initiated and a pulse obtained.

His vital signs now include a blood pressure of 70 by palpation and a pulse rate of 60; he is being ventilated with a bag-valve mask.

30. What size endotracheal tube will be needed to intubate this child?

  0   A. 6.0 cuffed tube
  0   B. 2.5 uncuffed tube
  0   C. 7.0 uncuffed tube
  0   D. 4.5 uncuffed tube

31. The child's vital signs suggest that the child may be suffering from:
    - 0 A. Anaphylactic shock
    - 0 B. Cardiogenic shock
    - 0 C. Spinal shock
    - 0 D. Septic shock

32. The collaborative emergency management of the patient in spinal shock would include:
    - 0 A. Administration of Ringer's lactate solution until the child's blood pressure is 80 systolic.
    - 0 B. Administration of packed red blood cells until the child's blood pressure is 80 systolic
    - 0 C. Administration of ceftriaxone intravenously to prevent meningitis
    - 0 D. Administration of a vasopressor intravenously until vasomotor control is restored

33. The initial emergency nursing care of this patient should be based on which of the following nursing diagnoses?
    - 0 A. Injury, potential for
    - 0 B. Tissue perfusion, altered (cerebral)
    - 0 C. Growth and development, altered
    - 0 D. Unilateral neglect

· · ·

34. An 8-year-old girl who has been diagnosed as having a concussion is going to be discharged from the emergency department. After having been given discharge instructions, her parents should be able to evaluate their daughter for what changes?
    - 0 A. Changes in blood pressure
    - 0 B. Changes in level of consciousness
    - 0 C. Changes in hemoglobin and hematocrit
    - 0 D. Changes in urinary output

A 27-year-old construction worker fell 3 feet from a ladder, landing on his buttocks, prior to his arrival in the emergency department. He comes into the emergency department walking, but complaining of pain in his lower back that is radiating down his legs. The only obvious signs of trauma are abrasions and bruising on his buttocks.

35. The initial assessment of this patient should include a history of:
    - 0 A. Loss of consciousness
    - 0 B. Tetanus immunization

   0 C. Pulmonary disease
   0 D. Diabetes

36. An important intervention for the patient who has fallen and sustained a back injury is:
   0 A. Obtaining a blood alcohol determination
   0 B. Obtaining an urinalysis
   0 C. Obtaining a bone profile
   0 D. Obtaining a drug screen

37. No acute injury was found in this patient. Based on his initial complaint, which of the following nursing diagnoses should the emergency nurse use for basing care?
   0 A. Fluid volume deficit
   0 B. Pain (acute)
   0 C. Cardiac output, decreased
   0 D. Infection, potential for

38. The patient is given discharge instructions for a low back injury. It is important that the emergency nurse question the patient about his understanding concerning which of the following possible signs of serious complications related to low back injury?
   0 A. Presence of some pain for 7 to 10 days
   0 B. Presence of soreness and stiffness in the lower back
   0 C. Presence of progressive weakness and bladder dysfunction
   0 D. Decrease in pain and stiffness

ANSWERS

1. **B. Intervention.** Diazepam crosses the blood-brain barrier more quickly than phenytoin or phenobarbital sodium. The appropriate dose of diazepam (Valium) for anticonvulsant therapy is 5 to 10 mg IV, which may be repeated at 10- to 15-minute intervals as needed for a total of not more than 30 mg. Signs and symptoms of respiratory depression must be carefully assessed.[3]
2. **A. Assessment.** It is easy to assume that this patient's seizures are being caused by alcohol intoxication, alcohol withdrawal, or not taking his medication properly. However, it is important to rule out a history of recent trauma, because the alcoholic patient is prone to the development of intracerebral bleeding more frequently following an injury.[4]
3. **C. Analysis.** Because the patient is having a seizure, he is unable to

maintain his airway. Even though the patient is at risk for injury, the emergency nurse's initial care should be directed at stabilizing the patient's airway. Related factors contributing to this nursing diagnosis include an increase in secretions and cognitive impairment.[5]

4. **B. Evaluation.** The toxic side effects of phenytoin are cardiac dysrhythmia, including bradycardia and heart block.[3]

5. **C. Assessment.** A fall may indicate that the seizure is possibly from trauma and not a medical cause.[6]

6. **D. Intervention.** Studies have demonstrated that the intraosseous route is comparable to giving the drug through an IV line. The other routes could be used, but the patient's response would be much slower.[7,8] An additional route (rectal) for diazepam has been evaluated in Europe and Canada, but rectal diazepam has not at the present time been approved by the Food and Drug Administration in this country.[9]

7. **C. Analysis.** One of the related factors contributing to this nursing diagnosis is an altered oxygen supply. During the seizure activity gas exchange may be impaired by airway obstruction and central nervous system depression.[5]

8. **A. Evaluation.** The most common side effects of this drug are drowsiness, lethargy, and depression. It is important to point this out to the child's parents. These effects will generally decrease after continued therapy.[3]

9. **C. Assessment.** Signs and symptoms associated with migraine headaches are many and varied. Visual disturbances, including homonymous hemianopsia, transient blindness, and photophobia, are seen. Other signs and symptoms include nausea and vomiting, vertigo, chills, cold hands and feet, abdominal distention, and cardiac dysrhythmia. However, unilateral pupillary changes and seizures would more likely suggest an expanding lesion.[10]

10. **A. Assessment.** Performing a baseline neurological assessment is imperative in the initial evaluation of a patient who is complaining of a severe headache. It is important to evaluate the patient for focal neurological signs and symptoms that could indicate an expanding lesion that would require immediate neurosurgical evaluation and intervention.[10]

11. **D. Intervention.** Dihydroergotamine, which is a semisynthetic derivative of ergot alkaloid, has been found to be effective in the acute management of migraine headaches. Because it is more rapid acting than ergotamine, it can offer the patient quicker pain relief. Meperidine and other opiates are not as effective as dihydroergotamine in treating patients suffering pain from severe migraine headaches, because these patients generally have a depletion of serotonin, which is required for opiates to be effective.[11]

12. **B. Intervention.** Application of a cold cloth, along with the prescribed

medical regimen, has been found to be helpful in the care of the patient with a headache. In addition, placing the patient in a quiet, dimly lit environment can also help decrease headache pain.[10]

13. **C. Analysis.** The emergency nursing care for the patient with a headache would include helping the patient with the management of his or her acute pain. Defining characteristics of pain include a verbal report of intense pain experience, narrowed focus, restlessness, unusual posture, diaphoresis, and increased muscle tension.[5]

14. **B. Evaluation.** IV prochlorperazine can cause postural hypotension because of its adrenergic blocking activity. The patient should be kept supine while in the emergency department and evaluated for postural hypotension before leaving the emergency department.[3,10]

15. **D. Assessment.** The motor function of the fifth cranial nerve (trigeminal) allows the patient to open and close his jaw. The sensory function of the fifth cranial nerve allows the patient to identify sharp and dull sensation on the forehead and cheek. The motor function of the seventh cranial nerve (facial) allows movement of the face, scalp, and eyelids. The sensory function of the seventh cranial nerve allows the patient taste for the anterior two thirds of the tongue.[4]

16. **B. Intervention.**

17. **A. Analysis.** While he is in the emergency department, the acute care of this patient should be based on the nursing diagnosis of tissue perfusion, altered (cerebral). The emergency nurse should be assessing the patient for changes in neurological status, as well as indications of increasing ICP, which would require acute interventions to prevent any further neurological injury to the patient.[5]

18. **B. Evaluation.** A major complication of heparin administration is acute bleeding. The emergency nurse should perform a hemotest on any emesis or stool and dipstick test on any urine after initiation of the heparin drip.[3]

19. **A. Assessment.** Because of the history given by the child's parents and based on the initial vital signs of the child, the emergency nurse should highly suspect that the child may be suffering from meningitis. Kernig's and Brudzinski's signs indicate meningeal irritation. The test for Kernig's sign is performed while the patient is lying flat. The patient's leg is flexed and then extended. If pain is elicited by this maneuver, meningeal irritation is indicated. Brudzinski's sign is elicited by flexing the patient's neck forward. Again, pain with this movement indicates meningeal irritation.[4]

20. **C. Intervention.** From the initial vital signs obtained, it is obvious that the child is in shock. It is probable that it is septic shock. The initial care

of the child should thus be directed at correcting his shock state. Administration of antibiotics and a lumbar puncture may be indicated later, but the initial emergency nursing interventions need to be based on stabilizing the patient's airway, breathing, and circulation.[12]

21. **B. Assessment.** The child's pH of 7.15 and HCO_3 of 18 indicate metabolic acidosis. In addition, the PCO_2 of 20 indicates that the child is hyperventilating in an attempt to compensate for this metabolic state.

22. **B. Analysis.** Defining characteristics of fluid volume deficit include hypotension, increased pulse rate, narrowed pulse pressure, and decreased urinary output.[5]

23. **A. Evaluation.** Adequate fluid resuscitation for a 3-year-old would be indicated with a urinary output of greater than 1 ml/kg per hour.[13]

24. **B. Assessment.** Basilar skull fractures occur at the base of the skull. They are not usually seen on x-ray examination but are diagnosed clinically. The signs of a basilar skull fracture are periorbital ecchymosis (raccoon's eyes), rhinorrhea, and otorrhea.[14]

25. **A. Assessment.** Additional indications of a skull fracture include a unilateral or bilateral hemotympanic membrane, mastoid ecchymosis (Battle's sign), and conjunctival hemorrhage without evidence of direct trauma to the eye(s).[14]

26. **C. Intervention.** When a basilar skull fracture occurs, the cribriform plate of the ethmoid bone may be fractured. This could potentially allow passage of such things as nasogastric tubes directly into the brain.[14]

27. **A. Intervention.** Mannitol is given to the adult patient in dosages of 1 to 2 g/kg body weight. Mannitol is generally infused over a period of 30 to 90 minutes.[3]

28. **A. Assessment.** Intracranial pressure is the result of the volume of brain tissue plus the volume of blood plus the volume of cerebrospinal fluid.[4]

29. **B. Analysis.** The appearance of pink, frothy sputum may indicate neurogenic pulmonary edema. These excessive secretions could potentially interfere with the patient's ability to be oxygenated. A related factor contributing to this nursing diagnosis is alveolar capillary membrane changes.[5]

30. **D. Intervention.** The formula that can be used to determine the appropriate tube size needed is 16 plus the age in years divided by 4. This would give an approximate size of 4.5. Other measures that can be used to estimate tube size include looking at the size of the child's little finger or nasal opening. It is important to note that an uncuffed tube should be used for a 2-year-old child.[7]

31. **C. Assessment.** Hypotension and bradycardia in a patient after a traumatic injury indicate that the patient may be in spinal shock. In addition, a child will normally be tachycardiac. In this case the child's pulse is 60 instead of 100. Spinal shock results when there is an injury or edema that blocks the sympathetic outflow tract, causing disruption of the vasomoter center, which causes loss of sympathetic tone.[15]

32. **D. Intervention.** Because the patient has suffered an injury that compromises his ability to control vasomotor tone, vasopressors are needed. Some of the drugs that are used include dopamine, norepinephrine, isoproterenol, and dobutamine.[14] Recent research has demonstrated that high-dose methylprednisone is an important adjunct in the treatment of spinal cord injury. This is used in both adult and pediatric patients.[16] The initial dosage of the drug is 30 mg/kg body weight diluted in normal saline and infused over a period of 15 minutes.[16]

33. **B. Analysis.** The initial care of this child should be based on providing both nursing and medical interventions to treat the complications of spinal shock and to prevent further injury. Defining characteristics of this nursing diagnosis include hypotension, decreased capillary filling, and alteration in mental status.[5]

34. **B. Evaluation.** Since the child has suffered a concussion, the child's parents need to know the signs and symptoms of possible neurological compromise following injury. The initial sign or symptom of neurological compromise is a change in mental status. It is important that the emergency nurse instruct the family on what to look for and be sure that the family understands the importance of this assessment.

35. **A. Assessment.** For any patient who has fallen and sustained possible neurological or spinal injury, a history of whether there was a loss of consciousness should be obtained. This would alert the emergency nurse to the possibility of any additional injury or injuries.[4]

36. **B. Intervention.** When a patient has sustained a fall resulting in back pain, the possibility of renal injury needs to be evaluated. This is done by obtaining a urine specimen and submitting it for urinalysis or using a dipstick to determine the presence of blood.[17]

37. **B. Analysis.** Because of the muscle spasms and tenderness that have resulted from the fall, the patient's care will need to be directed at relieving the acute pain he is suffering. Pain management may include prescribed medications, the use of hot or cold compresses, and bed rest.[17]

38. **C. Evaluation.** A serious complication of low back injury would be a disk herniation. Signs and symptoms of this complication include progressive weakness and bladder dysfunction.[17]

REFERENCES

1. Gress D: Recent advances in the evaluation and treatment of head and spine trauma, *Emerg Care Q* 5:15-23, 1989.
2. Tepas J et al: Mortality and head injury: the pediatric perspective, *J Pediatr Surg* 25:92-96, 1990.
3. Karb VB, Queener SF, Freeman JB: *Handbook of drugs for nursing practice,* St Louis, 1989, Mosby–Year Book.
4. Rudy E: *Advanced neurological and neurosurgical nursing,* St Louis, 1984, Mosby–Year Book.
5. McFarland GK, McFarlane EA: *Nursing diagnosis and intervention: planning for patient care,* St Louis, 1989, Mosby–Year Book.
6. Strange G: Febrile seizures: evaluation and management. In Barkin RM, editor: *The emergently ill child,* Rockville, Md, 1987, Aspen.
7. Chameides L: *Textbook of pediatric advanced life support,* Dallas, 1988, American Heart Association.
8. Manley L, Haley K, Dick M: Intraosseous infusion: rapid vascular access for critically ill or injured infants and children, *JEN* 14:63-69, 1988.
9. Rectal diazepam for acute seizures, *Emerg Med,* pp 35-38, 1990.
10. Fitzsimmons L: Migraine headache: recent concepts, *Top Emerg Med* 11:43-50, 1989.
11. Fitzsimmons L, Hadley S: Pharmacologic aspects of migraine therapy in the emergency department, *Top Emerg Med* 11:37-42, 1989.
12. Schonfeld N: Meningitis. In Barkin RM, editor: *The emergently ill child,* Rockville, Md, 1987, Aspen.
13. Mayer T: *Emergency management of pediatric trauma,* Philadelphia, 1985, WB Saunders.
14. Cardona V et al: *Trauma nursing from resuscitation through rehabilitation,* Philadelphia, 1988, WB Saunders.
15. Rea R, editor: *Trauma nursing core course,* Chicago, 1987, Emergency Nurses Association.
16. Bulletin from *JAMA,* Feb 1990.
17. Stine R, Marcus R: *A practical approach to emergency medicine,* Boston, 1987, Little, Brown.

Chapter 9 _____

Obstetrical Emergencies

REVIEW OUTLINE

I. Anatomy
   A. Aorta
   B. Ovarian artery
   C. Sigmoid colon
   D. Appendix
   E. Fallopian tubes
   F. Ovaries
   G. Uterus
   H. Vagina
   I. Labia
   J. Rectum
   K. Perineum
   L. Meatus
   M. Urethra
   N. Bladder
II. Physiology
   A. Menstrual cycle
   B. Stages of labor
   C. Ectopic pregnancy
   D. Disseminated intravascular coagulation (DIC)
   E. Prepartum and postpartum hemorrhage
III. Collaborative care of the patient with an obstetrical emergency
   A. Assessment
      1. ABCs (airway, breathing, circulation)
      2. History related to chief complaint
      3. Last menstrual period
      4. Estimated date of confinement
      5. Vaginal discharge and/or bleeding

6. Para, gravida, abortions
7. Abdominal tenderness
8. Height of the fundus
9. Ultrasound
10. Beta human chorionic gonadotropin (BHCG), complete blood cell count (CBC), type and screen or crossmatch

B. Interventions
   1. ABCs
   2. Transfusions
   3. Medications
   4. Emergency delivery
   5. Perimortem cesarean section
   6. APGAR scoring
   7. Neonatal resuscitation based on PALS (pediatric advanced life support)
   8. Measurement of fetal heart tones
   9. Dilation and curettage
   10. Culdocentesis
   11. Ultrasound
   12. Grief counseling

IV. Related nursing diagnoses
  A. Anxiety
  B. Family processes, altered
  C. Fluid volume deficit
  D. Grieving, anticipatory
  E. Infection, potential for
  F. Injury, potential for
  G. Pain
  H. Spiritual distress (distress of the human spirit)
  I. Trauma, potential for

V. Obstetrical emergencies
  A. Ectopic pregnancy
  B. Abortion
    1. Spontaneous
    2. Threatened
    3. Incomplete
    4. Septic
    5. Missed
  C. Hydatidiform mole
  D. Hyperemesis gravidarum

E. AIDS in the pregnant patient
F. Abruptio placentae
G. Placenta previa
H. Pregnancy-induced hypertension
    1. Preeclampsia
    2. Eclampsia
    3. Chronic hypertension
I. Emergency delivery
J. Perimortem cesarean section
K. Neonatal resuscitation
L. Maternal trauma

INTRODUCTION

When caring for the patient who is suffering from an obstetrical emergency, the emergency nurse needs to consider some important points. Pregnancy has a physiological impact on a woman that will influence her response to both trauma and other disease states. The pregnant patient will experience changes in her cardiovascular, pulmonary, and nervous systems. Pregnancy may alter the pattern or the severity of trauma or disease states; pregnancy may alter laboratory results; and pregnancy can have its own complications, such as abruptio placentae, amniotic fluid embolism, or eclampsia.[1]

Emergency births are obstetrical emergencies that cause increased excitement in the emergency department. The emergency nurse needs to be familiar with the care of the delivering mother, as well as with the initial resuscitation and stabilization of the infant. The *Pediatric Advanced Life Support* course available from the American Heart Association provides in-depth information related to the resuscitation of the neonate.

Finally, the care of the patient who is suffering from an obstetrical emergency can be very stressful for the patient, her family, and the emergency department staff. Unfortunately, many women suffer a miscarriage while in the emergency department, or they may lose their child as a result of abdominal trauma. Helping the family to deal with the sudden loss of their child can be very difficult. The emergency nurse needs to be aware of support sources for the patient and for the emergency department staff, as well.

The care of specific obstetrical emergencies is based on the particular emergency the patient is experiencing. The care of these patients needs to be appropriate and organized so that both the mother and the child may benefit.

REVIEW QUESTIONS
Vaginal Bleeding in Pregnancy

A 23-year-old woman who is 28 weeks pregnant comes to the emergency department complaining of vaginal bleeding that started 1 hour earlier.

1. Of the following, which is the most important piece of information the triage nurse should collect during the initial assessment of this patient?
   0 A. The date and description of her last menstrual period
   0 B. Whether she has been nauseated and vomiting over the past week
   0 C. Whether she is having any abdominal pain with the bleeding
   0 D. The number of children she has living with her at home

2. The emergency nurse should prepare the patient for all of the following procedures *except:*
   0 A. Insertion of a large-bore IV needle
   0 B. An ultrasound examination to evaluate the fetus
   0 C. Type and crossmatch for possible blood loss
   0 D. Pelvic examination by the emergency physician

3. The patient with severe vaginal bleeding related to either placenta previa or abruptio placentae is at risk for developing:
   0 A. Disseminated intravascular coagulation
   0 B. Adult respiratory distress syndrome
   0 C. Pregnancy-induced hypertension
   0 D. Trauma from delivery

4. The patient's initial vital signs are blood pressure, 80/40; pulse, 120; and respiratory rate, 23. The appropriate nursing diagnosis on which to plan this patient's care is:
   0 A. Airway clearance, ineffective, related to the patient's respiratory rate
   0 B. Fluid volume deficit related to vaginal bleeding
   0 C. Grieving, anticipatory, related to potential loss of pregnancy
   0 D. Infection, potential for, related to retained products of conception

5. For the patient at risk for DIC following blood loss, the emergency nurse should monitor the following:
   0 A. White blood cell count
   0 B. Rh factor
   0 C. Hemoglobin and hematocrit
   0 D. Platelet count

Ectopic Pregnancy

A 19-year-old woman comes to the emergency department complaining of left-sided abdominal pain. She states that it has been over 6 weeks since her last menstrual period and that she has had some spotting over the past few days. The patient is pale and diaphoretic.

6. The triage nurse places the patient in a pelvic examination room. The primary nurse should perform which of the following interventions during the initial assessment of this patient?
   0 A. Obtain orthostatic vital signs
   0 B. Perform a five-part neurological assessment
   0 C. Measure the patient's peak flow
   0 D. Ask the patient when she last ate and/or drank

7. The patient is complaining of pain in her left shoulder. This sign, associated with intraperitoneal bleeding, is known as:
   0 A. Kernig's sign
   0 B. Kehr's sign
   0 C. Homans' sign
   0 D. Brudzinski's sign

8. The emergency nurse should have which of the following laboratory studies done for this patient?
   0 A. Renal profile
   0 B. BHCG
   0 C. Hepatic profile
   0 D. Drug screen

9. The patient is diagnosed as having an ectopic pregnancy. While the nurse is preparing the patient for surgery, she begins to cry and states that she does not want to lose her baby. The emergency nurse should base the nursing care on which of the following nursing diagnoses?
   0 A. Spiritual distress (distress of the human spirit)
   0 B. Grieving, anticipatory
   0 C. Grieving, dysfunctional
   0 D. Thought processes, altered

10. The patient demonstrates acceptance of the need for her surgery, even though there will be a loss, by:
   0 A. Signing out against medical advice, stating that she will be all right once she gets home

0 B. Refusing to talk to her family when they enter the room
0 C. Stating that she knows that she will die if she does not have surgery
0 D. Stating that she will never get pregnant again if she consents to this surgery

Pregnancy-Induced Hypertension

A 34-year-old woman who is a gravida of 4 and a para of 3 is brought to the emergency department by the paramedics. She has been nauseated, vomiting, and complaining of a headache with blurred vision for 3 days. There have been no problems with her pregnancy until now. Her blood pressure is 160/110, her pulse is 110, and her respiratory rate is 20.

11. The diagnosis of preeclampsia has been made. The emergency nurse should continually assess this patient for signs and symptoms of:
    0 A. Seizures
    0 B. Pulmonary emboli
    0 C. Renal failure
    0 D. Congestive heart failure

12. The patient's blood pressure continues to go up. She is now irritable, complaining of severe pain in her head and in her upper right quadrant. The patient has bilateral clonus. The drug that the patient will receive is:
    0 A. Phenytoin, 1 to 5 g in 250 ml of normal saline
    0 B. Lorazepam, 3 to 5 mg IV push
    0 C. Magnesium sulfate, 4 to 6 g in 250 ml of normal saline
    0 D. Fentanyl, 2 to 5 ml IV push

13. A magnesium sulfate infusion is begun. The emergency nurse should evaluate which of the following as a symptom of toxicity?
    0 A. Normal deep tendon reflexes
    0 B. Urinary output greater than 30 ml/hr
    0 C. Magnesium level of 4 to 7 mEq/L
    0 D. Respiratory rate of less than 10

14. The patient is placed in a quiet room with dimmed lights. The side rails are padded and up on all sides of the bed. The patient's room is within sight of the nurse's station. These interventions are derived from which of the following nursing diagnoses?
    0 A. Infection, potential for

0   B. Thought processes, altered
0   C. Injury, potential for
0   D. Knowledge deficit

The Pregnant Trauma Patient

A 22-year-old woman who is 8 months pregnant has been involved in a motor vehicle crash. She was an appropriately restrained passenger (shoulder and lap belt) whose side of the car was struck by another vehicle going approximately 50 miles per hour. The patient is brought to the emergency department by helicopter with full cervical spine immobilization. Her vital signs are blood pressure, 70/40; pulse rate, 160; and respiratory rate, 32.

15. The most common type of fracture found in the pregnant trauma patient is:
    0   A. A fractured pelvis
    0   B. Femur fractures
    0   C. Lower rib fractures
    0   D. Cervical spine fractures

16. When the mother has suffered a ruptured uterus as a result of blunt abdominal trauma, the infant may die because of:
    0   A. Abdominal trauma
    0   B. Head trauma
    0   C. Pelvic trauma
    0   D. Chest trauma

17. The primary survey of the pregnant trauma patient includes all of the following *except:*
    0   A. Airway assessment
    0   B. Assessment of breath sounds
    0   C. Assessment of fetal heart tones
    0   D. Circulatory assessment

18. In addition to fluid and blood resuscitation, what other intervention could the emergency nurse perform to help increase the patient's blood pressure?
    0   A. Place a trauma catheter in the patient's subclavian vein
    0   B. Position the patient on her right side
    0   C. Position the patient in a left lateral position
    0   D. Place the patient in Trendelenburg position

19. Because the diaphragm is elevated by a gravid uterus and decreases the mother's oxygen reserve, the mother and fetus are at risk for hypoxia. The emergency nurse would base the nursing care on which of the following nursing diagnoses?

0   A. Airway clearance, ineffective
0   B. Gas exchange, impaired
0   C. Fluid volume deficit
0   D. Mobility, impaired physical

•   •   •

20. The pregnant patient demonstrates knowledge about the prevention of blunt trauma during pregnancy by:

0   A. Proper use of her lap and shoulder harness throughout her pregnancy
0   B. Not wearing her seat belt when she is in her third trimester
0   C. Wearing only a lap belt when she is in her third trimester
0   D. Not driving at all while she is pregnant

Emergency Delivery

A 17-year-old teenager called her mother home from work when she delivered a 30-week fetus at home alone. The teenager's mother called the paramedics, who have brought the teenage mother and infant to the emergency department.

21. The mother's vital signs are stable on arrival. The emergency nurse should next assess:

0   A. The status of the placenta
0   B. Whether the patient has any vaginal tears
0   C. Whether the mother wants to breast-feed
0   D. The height of the fundus

22. The infant is cyanotic and making little respiratory effort. The paramedics have suctioned the infant's lungs, applied oxygen by mask, dried the infant, and attempted tactile stimulation to improve the infant's respiratory function. The emergency nurse should:

0   A. Prepare equipment for intubation
0   B. Give epinephrine through an umbilical catheter
0   C. Perform chest compressions
0   D. Bag-mask ventilate the infant's lungs with high-flow oxygen

23. Chest compressions should be performed on the newborn:

0   A. When the infant's pulse is less than 60 beats per minute

0   B. When the infant's pulse is greater than 80 beats per minute
0   C. When the infant's pulse is 160 beats per minute
0   D. After the infant has been given atropine

· · ·

24. A 20-year-old woman comes to the triage desk screaming that she is having her baby. The patient's husband states that the baby is late. The patient is crying, pale, and diaphoretic. The emergency nurse prepares for an emergency delivery. Which of the following nursing diagnoses would be appropriate?
0   A. Fluid volume deficit
0   B. Fear
0   C. Cardiac output, decreased
0   D. Social isolation

Abortion
25. The most common complication of a missed abortion is:
0   A. Sepsis
0   B. Pulmonary emboli
0   C. Clotting abnormalities
0   D. Infertility

ANSWERS
1. **C. Assessment.** An important piece of information to be collected during the initial assessment of this patient is her description of the bleeding. Vaginal bleeding during pregnancy can occur for multiple reasons, including placenta previa, abruptio placentae, and preterm labor. If the bleeding is associated with pain, a boardlike rigidity of the abdomen, and signs and symptoms of hemorrhagic shock, the patient may have an abruptio placentae. Painless vaginal bleeding (usually after 28 weeks of gestation) and uterine contractions are symptomatic of placenta previa.[2]
2. **D. Intervention.** The patient who has a placenta previa or abruptio placentae should not have a vaginal examination unless the appropriate physicians and nursing teams are available to manage the potential delivery that could occur.[1,2]
3. **A. Assessment.** Because of the potential for the mother to lose a large amount of blood from both of these conditions, the patient is at risk for developing DIC.[1,2]
4. **B. Analysis.** The patient's vital signs indicate that she is suffering from some type of shock. Her vaginal bleeding could be the source of her blood

loss. The initial care of this patient needs to be directed at identifying and treating her shock.[1,3]

5. **D. Evaluation.** For the patient at risk of developing DIC, the platelet count should be monitored by the emergency department nurse. For the patient who has developed DIC, there is a decreased fibrinogen level and platelet count, increased prothrombin time (PT), increased partial thromboplastin time (PTT), increased whole blood–clotting time, and fibrin degradation products.[1,2]

6. **A. Assessment.** Obtaining orthostatic vital signs will provide information about whether or not the patient is bleeding. Based on the patient's chief complaint, there is a possibility of a ruptured ectopic pregnancy. In any young woman with the complaint of abdominal pain and amenorrhea, the emergency nurse should suspect the possibility of an ectopic pregnancy and base the initial assessment of the patient on this suspicion.[4]

7. **B. Assessment.** When the patient has significant intraperitoneal bleeding, the pain in the patient's abdomen from this bleeding may radiate to either shoulder. This sign is known as Kehr's sign and has also been associated with splenic injury.[4]

8. **B. Intervention.** A BHCG is obtained, along with a CBC, because both contribute information about the patient's condition.[4] Several other disease states can "mimic" an ectopic pregnancy, including spontaneous abortion, ovarian cyst, pelvic inflammatory disease (PID), and appendicitis. Other tests used to differentiate the diagnosis of ectopic pregnancy include pelvic ultrasonography, the patient's complaint, and a serum pregnancy test.[1]

9. **B. Analysis.** The defining characteristics of this nursing diagnosis include the expression of distress because of a potential loss and the realization or resolution of an impending death or loss.[3]

10. **C. Evaluation.** By acknowledging that she would die if she did not have the surgery, the patient is in the stage of developing awareness related to her loss. The emergency nurse should encourage the patient to continue to discuss her feelings.[3]

11. **A. Assessment.** Because seizures are a frequent complication of preeclampsia, the patient needs to be continually assessed while in the emergency department for signs and symptoms of seizures.[2]

12. **C. Intervention.** Magnesium sulfate is given in a loading dose of 4 to 6 as a 10% solution in 250 ml of IV fluid. It is infused rapidly over 15 minutes.[2]

13. **D. Evaluation.** Magnesium toxicity can cause respiratory depression. Respiratory failure can occur with magnesium sulfate levels of 12 to 15 mEq/L.[2]

14. **C. Analysis.** One of the goals of the emergency nursing care for this patient would be to prevent the potential injuries that could occur from seizures, a potential complication of preeclampsia.[2,3]

15. **A. Assessment.** The most common type of fracture found in the pregnant trauma patient is a pelvic fracture. The most frequent mechanism that causes injury in the pregnant patient is the motor vehicle, which generally results in the patient suffering some type of blunt trauma.[1,5]

16. **B. Assessment.** When the mother suffers enough impact from blunt trauma to rupture her uterus, fetal death is usually the result of a skull fracture with intracranial hemorrhage.[5]

17. **C. Assessment.** Saving the life of the mother is the primary objective during the initial management of the pregnant trauma patient. If the mother does not survive, the possibility that the fetus may survive — particularly depending on the fetus's gestational age — is limited. Assessment of fetal heart tones is completed during the secondary survey after the primary assessment and stabilization.[5]

18. **C. Intervention.** Because the gravid uterus compresses the vena cava when the patient is on her back, the patient will experience supine hypotension. Supine hypotension, or vena cava syndrome, is the result of the gravid uterus compressing the vena cava and aorta. The patient should be placed on the left lateral side as soon as the cervical spine has been cleared. If the cervical spine has not been cleared, a sandbag can be placed under the right side of the backboard.[5]

19. **B. Analysis.** A defining characteristic of this nursing diagnosis is hypoxia. A related factor contributing to this nursing diagnosis is an altered oxygen supply.[3]

20. **A. Evaluation.** The most common cause of fetal death during pregnancy is death of the mother. Women need to be educated about the proper way to wear safety restraints while they travel. The proper way to wear a restraint while pregnant is as follows: the lap belt is worn across the pelvis, and the shoulder harness is worn between the breasts and off the shoulder.[5]

21. **A. Assessment.** The status of the placenta should be assessed once the mother's ABCs have been assessed. The delivery of the placenta is indicated by a lengthening of the cord and a gush of blood. Once the placenta has been delivered, the emergency nurse should place it in a basin or a plastic bag, label it with the patient's name, and send it with the mother to the obstetrical unit.[2,6]

22. **D. Intervention.** Using the inverted pyramid for neonatal resuscitation, the emergency nurse should try bag-mask ventilation with high-flow

oxygen. If this should fail to improve the infant's status, chest compressions would be indicated, followed by intubation and the administration of medications.[7]

23. **A. Intervention.** Chest compressions are performed on a newborn when the pulse rate is less than 60 beats per minute and when, despite adequate ventilation with 100% oxygen after 30 seconds, the infant's condition does not improve.[7]

24. **B. Analysis.** The defining characteristics of fear include apprehension, fright, and sympathetic stimulation (cardiovascular excitation, vasoconstriction, and pupil dilation). Related factors include environmental stimuli and knowledge deficit, or not being familiar with the events to come.[3]

25. **C. Evaluation.** Because of the retained products of conception, the patient is at risk of developing hypofibrinogenemia.[8]

REFERENCES

1. Reedy N, Brucker M: Obstetric and gynecologic emergencies. In Kitt S, Kaiser J, editors: *Emergency nursing: a physiologic and clinical perspective,* Philadelphia, 1990, WB Saunders.
2. Kostenbauder M: *Maternal-newborn nursing,* Springhouse, PA, 1989, Springhouse.
3. McFarland GK, McFarlane EA: *Nursing diagnosis and intervention: planning for patient care,* St Louis, 1989, Mosby–Year Book.
4. Dickinson E: Gynecological emergencies, *J Emerg Med Serv* 3:20-30, 1990.
5. Dees G, Fuller M: Blunt trauma in the pregnant patient, *JEN* 15:495-499, 1990.
6. Kozole A, Andrea J: Mock delivery: an educational tool for the emergency department, *JEN* 16:162-165, 1990.
7. Chameides L: *Textbook of pediatric advanced life support,* Dallas, 1988, American Heart Association.
8. Thomas HA, O'Connor R, Hoffman G: *Emergency medicine: self-assessment and review,* ed 2, St Louis, 1988, Mosby–Year Book.

Chapter 10

Ocular Emergencies

REVIEW OUTLINE

I. Anatomy and physiology
    A. Anatomical structures
        1. Anterior chamber
        2. Aqueous humor
        3. Canthus
        4. Central retinal artery
        5. Choroid
        6. Ciliary body
        7. Cornea
        8. Conjunctiva
        9. Crystalline lens
      10. Frontal bone
      11. Iris
      12. Lacrimal duct and glands
      13. Limbus
      14. Macula
      15. Maxilla
      16. Nasal bone
      17. Optic nerve
      18. Orbits
      19. Posterior chambers
      20. Punctum
      21. Pupil
      22. Sclera
      23. Sinuses
      24. Retina

        25. Tarsal plate

        26. Vitreous body

        27. Zygomatic bone

   B. Physiology

        1. Vision

        2. Accommodation

        3. Extraocular eye movements

II. Ocular assessment

   A. History of illness or injury

        1. Mechanism and time

        2. AMPLE history

           a. Allergies

           b. Medications

           c. Past medical history

           d. Last meal

           e. Events or treatment prior to arrival

        3. Change in condition from onset of symptoms to arrival in the emergency department

   B. Pain

        1. Provocation

        2. Quality

        3. Radiation

        4. Severity

        5. Time

   C. General appearance of eye

        1. Edema, erythema

        2. Bleeding, tearing, discharge

   D. Visual acuity

        1. Test with and without glasses or contact lenses

        2. Use a Snellen eye chart if possible

        3. Determine if the patient can see fingers if unable to see the eye chart; start at approximately 10 feet and see if the patient can count the number of fingers being held up; continue to move closer to the patient until the patient can see the fingers; this is recorded as "count fingers at X feet"; if the patient still cannot see fingers within 2 to 3 feet, determine if the patient can see hand motion; record as "hand motion at X feet"; if the patient has only light perception, use a penlight to see if the patient can determine which direction light is coming from

    4. Visual changes include:
      a. Blindness
      b. Blurring
      c. Diplopia
      d. Cloudy or smoky
      e. Photophobia

  E. Visual fields: face the patient; the patient and the examiner occlude opposite eyes; the examiner moves to bring his or her hands into the visual field from the periphery; assess all four quadrants; the absence of vision in any quadrant is recorded

  F. Extraocular eye motion (EOM): face the patient; have the patient focus on an object such as a pencil; move the pencil up, down, to the left, and to the right; observe the patient's ability to move the eyes equally in all directions

  G. Pupil reactivity: test for direct and consensual pupillary response when light is shone in the eye

  H. Pupil accommodation: have the patient focus on a near and then distant object; accommodation causes convergence of the eyes and pupillary constriction

  I. Past medical history
    1. Glaucoma
    2. Chronic eye disease, past eye trauma
    3. Diabetes
    4. Cardiovascular disease
    5. Hypertension

III. Diagnostic studies or procedures
  A. Tonometry
  B. Fluorescein stain
  C. Slit-lamp examination
  D. Laboratory
  E. Radiology
  F. Visual acuity charts

IV. Related nursing diagnoses
  A. Anxiety
  B. Fear
  C. Knowledge deficit
  D. Pain
  E. Sensory/perceptual alterations (visual)
  F. Tissue perfusion, altered (optic nerve)

INTRODUCTION

Ocular trauma is a common occurrence. The American Academy of Ophthalmology estimates that approximately 1.5 million eye injuries occur yearly.[1] Eye injuries may be caused by blunt or penetrating trauma. Blunt trauma most frequently is the result of physical violence secondary to altercations. Penetrating trauma is usually caused by industrial accidents but may also be the result of an assault. Both blunt and penetrating trauma may be caused by motor vehicle accidents, sports-related injuries, or falls.

Millions of Americans suffer from chronic eye disease. They, too, may be seen in the emergency department with an exacerbation of an existing illness.

Whether the patient has a traumatic or a medical emergency, the emergency nurse must rapidly assess the situation and intervene to prevent permanent visual loss. Patients will have anxiety because of a fear of disfigurement and/or loss of vision. Therefore the emergency nurse must also be skilled in providing emotional support, as well as physical care.

REVIEW QUESTIONS
Infection

Mr. Lord, a 22-year-old construction worker, comes to the emergency department with complaints of pain, redness, and drainage in the left eye, which has worsened over the past 2 days. He is diagnosed as having conjunctivitis.

1. Conjunctivitis is an inflammation of the conjunctiva that may be caused by:
   0   A. A bacterial infection
   0   B. A viral infection
   0   C. Allergies
   0   D. All of the above

2. On assessment of Mr. Lord's visual acuity, the emergency nurse would expect to find:
   0   A. A decrease in visual acuity in the affected eye
   0   B. A decrease in visual acuity in both eyes
   0   C. No change in the patient's visual acuity
   0   D. An improvement in visual acuity in both eyes

3. An appropriate nursing diagnosis for the patient with conjunctivitis would be:

0   A. Sensory/perceptual alterations (input deficit)
0   B. Infection, potential for
0   C. Pain
0   D. Tissue perfusion, altered (optic nerve)

4. Initial nursing interventions for Mr. Lord should be aimed at providing comfort. One method for this would include:
0   A. Providing cold compresses to the affected eye
0   B. Providing warm compresses to the affected eye
0   C. Not providing any compresses, since they only irritate the eye further
0   D. Irrigating the affected eye with warm saline

5. When providing direct care to Mr. Lord's eye, the nurse should wear gloves:
0   A. For self-protection
0   B. To protect Mr. Lord's nonaffected eye
0   C. To protect other patients
0   D. All of the above

6. To evaluate the effectiveness of nursing interventions directed toward pain relief, the nurse would expect to see Mr. Lord:
0   A. Pacing in his room
0   B. Sitting in the chair, tapping his feet, and holding the affected eye
0   C. Sitting in the chair in a relaxed body position
0   D. Lying on the stretcher in a fetal position and rocking his head in his hands

Trauma

Mr. Gordon, an 18-year-old man, comes to the emergency department with the chief complaint of eye pain as a result of an altercation. Mr. Gordon states that he was punched in the eye by his enemy's fist. On medical evaluation, he is diagnosed as having a hyphema. Usually the product of blunt trauma, a hyphema is bleeding from the vessels of the iris into the anterior chamber.

7. Assessment findings associated with a hyphema include:
0   A. Normal visual acuity
0   B. Pain
0   C. Hemorrhage from the inner canthus
0   D. All of the above

8. An appropriate nursing diagnosis for Mr. Gordon would be:
   - 0   A.   Social isolation
   - 0   B.   Pain (acute)
   - 0   C.   Fluid volume deficit, potential
   - 0   D.   Airway clearance, ineffective

9. Interventions for Mr. Gordon include proper patient positioning once his cervical spine has been cleared. Mr. Gordon should:
   - 0   A.   Lie flat
   - 0   B.   Sit upright
   - 0   C.   Recline, turned on the affected side, with the head of the bed at 45 degrees
   - 0   D.   Recline, turned on the unaffected side, with the head of the bed at 45 degrees

10. Nursing interventions are also aimed at protecting the eye from further injury while the patient is in the emergency department. This can be accomplished by:
    - 0   A.   Patching the affected eye
    - 0   B.   Patching both eyes
    - 0   C.   Covering the affected eye with a metal shield
    - 0   D.   Covering both eyes with a metal shield

11. Mr. Gordon is given an analgesic and is awaiting admission to the hospital for observation of the eye injury. The emergency nurse should periodically evaluate Mr. Gordon to assess that the hyphema has not worsened. Evaluation criteria would include:
    - 0   A.   A decrease in visual acuity
    - 0   B.   No change in blurring of vision
    - 0   C.   Layered blood visualized in the anterior chamber increases from filling one third to one half of the anterior chamber
    - 0   D.   A. change in his level of consciousness

Spontaneous Eye Pain

Mr. Thomas, a 66-year-old man, comes to the emergency department with complaints of a severe headache located along the left eyebrow. He states that he can barely see out of his left eye and that when he looks toward the lights, he sees halos. Mr. Thomas denies head trauma and states that these symptoms began about 1 hour earlier.

12. The emergency nurse suspects Mr. Thomas has:
    - 0   A.   Blepharitis

0   B. Retinal detachment
0   C. Central retinal artery occlusion
0   D. Acute, narrow-angle glaucoma

13. Several classic assessment findings will assist the emergency medical team in their diagnosis of acute, narrow-angle glaucoma. The affected eye's pupil will be:
0   A. Semidilated, nonreactive
0   B. Dilated, yet reactive
0   C. Constricted, nonreactive
0   D. Normal

14. On palpation, the affected eye will feel:
0   A. Rock-hard
0   B. Soft and mushy
0   C. Like rubber
0   D. Normal

15. An appropriate nursing diagnosis for Mr. Thomas would be:
0   A. Anxiety
0   B. Pain
0   C. Sensory/perceptual alterations (visual)
0   D. All of the above

16. Mr. Thomas is given an analgesic for pain. Anticipatory care would also dictate that Mr. Thomas be given an:
0   A. Antibiotic
0   B. Antiemetic
0   C. Antiinflammatory
0   D. Anticoagulant

17. Mr. Thomas is given an osmotic diuretic. The rationale for this therapy for the patient with acute, narrow-angle glaucoma is that the diuretic will:
0   A. Lower intraocular pressure
0   B. Prevent cerebral edema
0   C. Raise mean arterial pressure
0   D. Improve cardiac output

18. Mr. Thomas is also given 4% pilocarpine. What criteria should the nurse use to evaluate the effectiveness of this drug?
0   A. An increase in intraocular pressure

0   B. An increase in visual acuity

0   C. An increase in blurred vision

0   D. An increase in halos seen around lights

19. Mr. Thomas's "attack" is broken. His vital signs are stable, visual acuity has improved, and pain has substantially subsided. He is given discharge instructions and has an appointment to see an ophthalmologist the next day. Mrs. Thomas begins to cry and expresses fear that her husband has lost his vision forever. An appropriate reply would be:
0   A. Mr. Thomas's sight can return to normal with appropriate treatment
0   B. Mr. Thomas will probably go blind in the future, but many social programs can help them adjust to this change
0   C. Mr. Thomas will probably go blind in the affected eye only, which means only minimal changes in his daily routine
0   D. Mrs. Thomas should address these concerns with the ophthalmologist

Foreign Bodies

Mr. Roberts, a 24-year-old carpenter, comes to the emergency department with complaints of pieces of wood in his left eye. Several large foreign bodies are visible. The eye is reddened, tearing, and painful. Visual acuity is normal.

20. The first nursing intervention for Mr. Roberts should be to:
0   A. Irrigate the eye with normal saline
0   B. Manually remove the larger pieces of wood
0   C. Anesthetize the eye with the appropriate eye drops
0   D. Test Mr. Roberts's visual acuity

21. One would expect Mr. Roberts's visual acuity to be:
0   A. Decreased in the affected eye
0   B. Decreased in both eyes
0   C. Normal
0   D. Increased in the unaffected eye

22. It is determined that Mr. Roberts has sustained a corneal abrasion secondary to the foreign bodies. The affected eye is patched, and Mr. Roberts is provided with antibiotic ointment as well as instructions on how to apply the ointment. He is also instructed that his eye pain will return. The pain can be relieved by application of:
0   A. Warm compresses

0 B. A tight eye patch
0 C. A topical anesthetic
0 D. Over-the-counter eye drops

ANSWERS

1. **D. Assessment.** Conjunctivitis is caused by all the agents listed: bacteria, a virus, or allergies.
2. **C. Assessment.** The patient with conjunctivitis usually has no change in visual acuity.
3. **C. Analysis.** Mr. Lord does not have sensory/perceptual alterations, since his visual acuity is normal. He does not have the potential for infection, since he already has an infection. He does have pain.
4. **B. Intervention.** Providing warm compresses to the affected eye does provide comfort to the patient with conjunctivitis. Cold compresses provide comfort to the trauma patient by decreasing the development of periorbital edema.
5. **D. Intervention.** The nurse should wear gloves when providing care to anyone's eyes, since human tears have been demonstrated to harbor chlamydia, bacteria, herpes simplex virus, and the AIDS virus. Wearing gloves will protect the nurse and other patients the nurse may come in contact with, as well as the patient's nonaffected eye.
6. **C. Evaluation.** The patient's pain and eye irritation should subside with the appropriate interventions. Therefore the nurse should observe a calm, relaxed position.
7. **B. Assessment.** The patient with a hyphema will demonstrate a decrease in visual acuity in the affected eye and complain of pain, and a layer of blood will be observable in the anterior chamber of the eye.
8. **B. Analysis.** Mr. Gordon has pain, as stated in the case study.
9. **B. Intervention.** The patient with a hyphema should assume an upright position.
10. **C. Intervention.** The patient with a hyphema requires only a metal shield to protect the affected eye from further injury.
11. **B. Evaluation.** No change in blurring of vision will indicate that the hyphema has not worsened (i.e., bleeding into the anterior chamber has not increased). Both *A* and *C* would indicate that further bleeding into the anterior chamber has occurred.
12. **D. Assessment.** Mr. Thomas has classic symptoms of acute, narrow-angle glaucoma. Blepharitis is an inflammation of the eyelid margins and does not affect visual acuity. Retinal detachment is usually the result of trauma, although it can have medical causes. The patient with retinal detachment

will complain of seeing flashes of light (even with the eye closed), a shower of black dots in the peripheral vision, or a decrease in vision with a "curtain" blocking part of the visual field. Central retinal artery occlusion presents as a painless, sudden loss of vision, and the visual acuity is limited to light perception.

13. **A. Assessment.** The patient with acute, narrow-angle glaucoma will have a pupil that is semidilated and nonreactive.

14. **A. Assessment.** The patient with acute, narrow-angle glaucoma will have a globe that is rock-hard on palpation. The flow of aqueous humor from the posterior to the anterior chamber is blocked, causing an increase in intraocular pressure. Normal intraocular pressure is less than 20 mm Hg. The patient with acute, narrow-angle glaucoma may have an intraocular pressure as high as 60 mm Hg.

15. **D. Analysis.** All of the nursing diagnoses listed would be appropriate ones for Mr. Thomas.

16. **B. Intervention.** Patients with acute, narrow-angle glaucoma frequently experience severe nausea and vomiting. Anticipatory care would dictate the use of an antiemetic to decrease nausea and prevent vomiting.

17. **A. Intervention.** The use of an osmotic diuretic for the patient with acute, narrow-angle glaucoma serves to decrease intraocular pressure. Because diuretics "dehydrate" the body, the amount of aqueous humor produced will also hopefully be decreased, lowering the intraocular pressure.

18. **B. Evaluation.** The effectiveness of 4% pilocarpine eye drops can be evaluated by an increase or improvement in visual acuity. Pilocarpine constricts the pupil, pulling the iris away from the cornea and out of the angle, allowing for the free flow of aqueous humor from the posterior to the anterior chamber.

19. **A. Intervention.** Mr. Thomas's sight can return to normal with the appropriate treatment. Patients may be treated medically or may require a peripheral iridectomy. In this surgical procedure, a small opening is made at the periphery of the iris, providing an alternate path for the flow of aqueous humor. Acute, narrow-angle glaucoma presents a serious threat to the patient's vision if it is not treated within a few hours.

20. **C. Intervention.** Providing anesthetic drops is a nursing intervention with the appropriate standing orders. This should be a priority of care, since the patient will then be able to cooperate with all other procedures.

21. **C. Assessment.** With simple extraocular foreign bodies, the visual acuity should be normal to slightly abnormal. Visual acuity would be affected if a foreign body were intraocular.

22. **B. Intervention.** To alleviate his recurrent pain, Mr. Roberts should be

instructed to apply the antibiotic ointment as directed, double-patch the eye to achieve a tight eye patch, apply an ice pack, and use over-the-counter analgesics. The purpose of an eye patch is to protect the eye, absorb secretions, and promote comfort. A tight eye patch will act as a pressure dressing and will relieve pain, as well as promote healing. Patients should never be given a bottle of topical anesthetics, since they impair corneal healing and promote the development of corneal ulcers. Patients may also reinjure the eye without knowing it if they consistently use a topical anesthetic.

REFERENCE

1. Karesh JW: Ocular and periocular trauma, *Emerg Med Serv* 18(6):46-55, 1989.

ADDITIONAL READINGS

Bates B: *A guide to physical examination,* Philadelphia, 1983, JB Lippincott.

Goldman R: For your eyes only, *Emergency* 19 (12):27-29, 1987.

Kitt S, Kaiser J, editors: *Emergency nursing: a physiologic and clinical perspective,* Philadelphia, 1990, WB Saunders.

Knezevick BA: *Trauma nursing: principles and practice,* East Norwalk, Conn, 1986, Appleton-Century-Crofts.

Rea R et al: *Emergency nursing core curriculum,* ed 3, Philadelphia, 1987, WB Saunders.

Sheehy SB, Marvin JA, Jimmerson CL: *Manual of clinical trauma care: the first hour,* St Louis, 1989, Mosby–Year Book.

Chapter 11 _____

Organ Donation

REVIEW OUTLINE

I.   Anatomy and physiology
    A. Anatomy of organs and tissues involved in transplantation
        1. Cornea
        2. Kidney
        3. Skin
        4. Liver
        5. Heart
        6. Lung
        7. Pancreas
        8. Bone
        9. Heart for valves
      10. Bone, ligament
      11. Middle ear
    B. Physiological systems review
        1. Fluid and electrolytic balance
        2. Cardiac system
        3. Respiratory system
        4. Renal system
        5. Hepatic system
        6. Pancreatic system
        7. Neurological system
        8. Skeletal system
        9. Integumentary system
      10. Immunosuppression
II.   Assessment skills
    A. History
    B. In-depth head-to-toe physical assessment

III. Historical perspective
  A. Legislative issues
    1. Consolidated Omnibus Budget Reconciliation Act (COBRA), 1986
    2. Organ Donation Request Act, 1987
    3. Uniform Anatomical Gift Act
    4. State laws
      a. Routine referral
      b. Required request
    5. Hospital policy
    6. Emergency department policy
  B. Brain death
    1. Definition
    2. Criteria
    3. Brain death status
      a. State
      b. Federal
      c. Hospital policy
    4. Coroner's cases
IV. Identification of potential organ and tissue donors
  A. Respiratory (artificially maintained) and circulatory functions
  B. Tissue donation: either respiratory- and circulatory-maintained brain-dead patients or patients who have died of cardiorespiratory arrest
  C. Identification of potential donor
    1. Past medical history
    2. History of presenting injury or condition
    3. Present physiological condition
    4. Contraindications
    5. Brain death
  D. Organ procurement organization
    1. Protocols
    2. Role of coordinators
      a. With emergency department
      b. With families
      c. With donors
  E. Brain death
    1. Definition
      a. Generally accepted (Harvard)
      b. State
      c. Hospital policy

       2. Role of ethics committee

   F. Criteria for organ donor suitability

       1. Vary according to organ and/or tissue involved

       2. Time frames for retrievability

   G. Exclusionary criteria for donor identification

       1. Untreated septicemia

       2. AIDS

       3. Viral hepatitis

       4. Active tuberculosis

       5. Malignancy, except primary brain tumor

       6. Disease of the donated organ and/or tissue

       7. Chronic systemic disease

V.   Donor maintenance management

   A. Goal: ensure organ viability

       1. Maintain optimal hydration

       2. Maintain adequate oxygenation

       3. Maintain hemodynamic stability

          a. Maintain adequate fluid hydration (central venous pressure [CVP] 8 to 12 cm)

          b. Maintain urine output (>100 ml/hr)

          c. Maintain systolic blood pressure stability at >100 mm Hg

          d. Maintain electrolyte balance and blood glucose level

          e. Maintain normal body temperature

          f. Prevent and treat infection

   B. Basic principles of donor management

       1. Resuscitation

       2. Organ perfusion

       3. Hydration

       4. Diuretics

       5. Avoidance of infection

VI. Approaching families of potential donors

   A. Establishing legal next of kin

       1. Spouse

       2. Adult brother or sister

       3. Guardian

       4. Any other person authorized or under obligation to dispose of the body

   B. Approach to family: intervention

       1. Obligations to approach

       2. Dignified, professional manner

       3. Positive attitude

           4. Knowledgeable
           5. Offer emotional support
           6. Answer questions; allow expression of feelings
           7. Accept and support decision of family

   C. Involvement of others
           1. Physician
           2. Social worker
           3. Clergy
           4. Medical examiner and/or coroner
           5. Organ procurement coordinator

   D. Answers to most commonly asked questions
           1. No cost
           2. No disfigurement
           3. No disruption of funeral arrangements
           4. Confidentiality maintained
           5. Donated organs always given to those in great need
           6. Religious leaders support organ donations
           7. Family can visit patient's body

VII. Specific emergency nursing considerations
   A. Completing physical assessment
   B. Obtaining a history
   C. Awareness of organ and tissue donation inclusion and exclusion criteria
   D. Knowledge of appropriate ways to approach families
   E. Knowledge of brain death criteria
   F. Awareness of role of organ procurement coordinator
   G. Awareness of other support services personnel and referral agencies
   H. Knowledge about donor management protocols
   I. Awareness of legal next of kin
   J. Coordination with intensive care unit
           1. Donor maintenance
           2. Documenting, reporting
           3. Following policy and/or procedure
   K. Awareness of donor sources (organs, tissues)
           1. Heart
           2. Kidney
           3. Liver
           4. Pancreas
           5. Heart-lung
           6. Skin

       7. Bone, connective tissue
       8. Saphenous vein
       9. Middle ear
     10. Eye, cornea
     11. Heart for heart valves
     12. Bone marrow
  L. Legal issues
       1. Legal next of kin
       2. Obligation by law to ask
       3. Telephone consent (witnessed)
       4. Documentation
VIII. Related nursing diagnoses
  A. Breathing pattern, effective
  B. Cardiac output, decreased
  C. Coping, family: potential for growth
  D. Coping, ineffective family
  E. Fluid volume deficit, potential
  F. Gas exchange, impaired
  G. Grieving, anticipatory
  H. Infection, potential for
  I. Skin integrity, impaired
  J. Spiritual distress (distress of the human spirit)
  K. Tissue perfusion, altered
  L. Urinary elimination, altered patterns

INTRODUCTION

*T*here have been many advances in technology, technique, and immunosuppression to make transplantation successful. Organ supply, however, remains a major factor limiting organ transplantation,[1] and thousands of people await transplants. Two specific pieces of legislation mandate that hospitals and medical personnel inform all families of their option of organ and tissue donation. A brief overview of these laws is presented here. A discussion of the vital role emergency nurses play in identifying and maintaining potential donors follows.

    The first legislation, the Consolidated Omnibus Budget Reconciliation Act (COBRA), was passed in 1986. This became effective on Oct. 1, 1987, and made provisions requiring all hospitals receiving Medicaid or Medicare reimbursement to do the following: (1) have written protocols for donor identification, (2) inform families of their option of organ and tissue donation, (3) observe discretion and sensitivity, and (4) notify organ procurement organizations of potential organ or tissue donors.[2]

The federal government also enacted a second piece of legislation, the Organ Donation Request Act (the "required request" act), in January 1987 because health care professionals had demonstrated reluctance in asking families for organ and tissue donation. This act outlined the following provisions: (1) the next of kin must be asked for consent; (2) consent may be secured by the attending physician; (3) deference should be paid to the donor's religious beliefs; (4) notification must be made to the organ procurement organization; and (5) no sanctions for hospital noncompliance.[3]

These legislative acts make it clear that hospitals must comply with the provisions outlined, or Medicare and Medicaid reimbursement may be withheld. "Required request" laws now exist in all states and require hospitals to notify the nearest organ procurement agency when brain death is diagnosed and also require request for organ and tissue donation when the deceased meet specified criteria.

Local procurement agencies play a large role in assisting the emergency department nurse in complying with these laws. The local organ procurement agency is linked with the United Network for Organ Sharing System (UNOS) and by way of a national computer system connects with current information on all potential recipients and organs available. This system ensures that those with the greatest need receive organs and/or tissues first. The organ procurement agency serves a vital role in providing information and guidance to the emergency department nurse.

Since emergency department nurses are frequently the first health care professionals to identify a potential donor, they must be diligent in their efforts to identify and manage potential donors to help meet the increasing demand for organs and tissues. Although organ donors are usually transferred to the intensive care unit for maintenance until brain death has been declared and consent obtained from the family, the emergency department nurse provides emotional support for the family and provides proper nursing management of the patient prior to transport. Tissue donors may be identified and maintained in the emergency department, because no ventilatory or cardiovascular support is necessary. After the patient is determined to fit the criteria for organ and/or tissue donation, the emergency department nurse should follow the established protocol quickly and notify the local organ procurement organization.

Nurses can facilitate the decision making of families who are considering donation, and they can work with the health care team to provide the concept of organ donation to families who have not considered it at all. This is important, because although many families would be willing to donate organs for transplantation, most families will not think of donation unless someone cares enough to let them know about this opportunity. The experience of most organ procurement agencies has been that 80% to 85% of all families approached agree to donate their relative's organs in the hope of helping someone else.[4]

It is crucial that emergency department nurses know their state laws and hospital/departmental policies in relation to organ and tissue donation. They must be able to identify potential donors, know the role of the organ procurement agency, know the interventions to be used in the care of donor management, know how to approach families, and know the nursing diagnoses related to the care of these patients. Efforts to increase the number of available donor organs and tissues are underway to meet the steadily increasing demand. In addition, the emergency department nurse must become comfortable with approaching families and making a request. Increasing public awareness through education regarding the need to consider donation remains a role of the emergency department nurse.

REVIEW QUESTIONS

A 56-year-old man is brought to the emergency department by the rescue squad. He was on a construction site and had fallen from a bridge into a river. He has suffered severe head injuries and has fixed, dilated pupils. CPR was begun at the scene. The patient is brought to the emergency department under full CPR, which is unsuccessful.

1. The nurse, in collaboration with the physician, must determine if this patient is a potential organ/tissue donor. What is *most* important in determining if this patient is a potential organ/tissue donor?
   - 0   A. Completing a physical examination and obtaining a detailed history.
   - 0   B. Calling the organ procurement agency
   - 0   C. Asking the family for consent
   - 0   D. Notifying the coroner

2. Current federal and state laws require that:
   - 0   A. Families of all potential donors be asked for organ/tissue donation
   - 0   B. Families of all medically suitable donors be asked about the possibility of donation
   - 0   C. Only families who have no religious obligations be asked about organ/tissue donation
   - 0   D. Families never be asked about organ/tissue donation while the patient is still in the emergency department

3. The emergency department nurse finds the deceased patient's driver's license among his belongings. The patient had signed the donor card. When the family is approached about organ donation, the patient's relatives vehemently oppose the idea of donation. The Uniform Anatomical Gift Act allows for:

   0   A. The individual's decision to override the wishes of relatives
   0   B. Hospitals to create their own policies about organ/tissue donation
   0   C. The family's decision to override the patient's request
   0   D. The need to contact a judge before any decision can be made

4. When the family is told that CPR was ineffective and that the patient has died, the family members begin to yell and scream. One of them attempts to hit the emergency physician. Attempts to calm the family are to no avail. The nursing diagnosis on which the emergency nurse would base care is:

   0   A. Coping, ineffective family
   0   B. Family processes, altered
   0   C. Grieving, anticipatory
   0   D. Injury, potential for

5. Based on the family's reaction to the news of the loss of their family member, the best approach for the emergency nurse to use concerning organ/tissue donation would be to:

   0   A. Abstain from asking about organ donation because they are too upset
   0   B. Ask the family, and if they do not agree, try to convince them that they should donate
   0   C. Offer emotional support, such as from a chaplain, and when the family is calmer, offer them the option of donation
   0   D. Tell the family it is the nurse's job to ask them about organ donation

· · ·

6. The major goal in organ donation management is to:

   0   A. Reassure family members that the organs of the deceased are donated to the person of their choice
   0   B. Ensure organ viability
   0   C. Make sure the religious beliefs of the family are explored
   0   D. Notify the appropriate agencies

7. A recommended method of maintaining fluid volume in the patient who is a potential organ donor is to:

0   A. Slowly infuse dextrose 5% in water (D_5W)
0   B. Rapidly infuse normal saline or Ringer's lactate solution
0   C. Transfuse the patient with packed red blood cells
0   D. Begin a dopamine drip

8. If adequate fluid replacement therapy has been attempted and is unsuccessful, the best choice of vasopressors to be used to maintain a systolic blood pressure of greater than 100 mm Hg is:

0   A. Dopamine
0   B. Norepinephrine
0   C. Metaraminol bitartrate
0   D. Azathioprine

9. Organ donors are usually transferred to the intensive care unit until brain death is determined and the family has given consent for donation. The emergency department nurse has a major role in:

0   A. Identifying and stabilizing the condition of the patient who fits the donor criteria
0   B. Trying to convince the patient's family that they need to consent to donation because of the great need for donors
0   C. Explaining the concept of brain death to the family and what might happen to the patient in the intensive care unit
0   D. Determining when the patient has met brain death criteria

10. A 35-year-old single woman has been deemed an appropriate candidate for organ donation. The nurse approaches the waiting room and finds 12 of the patient's relatives there. The sister of the patient has become the spokesperson for the family. The emergency department nurse needs to determine who is the legal next of kin. Of the following, the nurse should obtain consent from the:

0   A. Patient's sister, since she is the spokesperson for the family
0   B. Patient's boyfriend
0   C. Mother of the patient
0   D. Woman who states she is the patient's closest friend

11. Which of the following is *not* an exclusionary criterion for organ donation?

0   A. AIDS
0   B. Hepatitis

0 C. Obesity

0 D. Active tuberculosis

12. Candidates for organ donation who are victims of drownings or, in the case of severe burns, who require prolonged ventilatory support have been thought to be less suitable for organ donation because of which of the following nursing diagnoses?

    0 A. Fluid volume deficit, potential, related to prolonged ventilatory support

    0 B. Infection, potential for, related to prolonged ventilatory support

    0 C. Poisoning, potential for, related to prolonged ventilatory support

    0 D. Breathing pattern, ineffective, related to ventilatory support

ANSWERS

1. **A. Assessment.** A thorough history and physical examination are essential to the initial assessment of donor suitability. A number of underlying conditions immediately exclude the potential donor from further consideration.[2,4,5]

2. **A. Intervention.** The law requires that *all* potential donors (or their families) be approached. Families may wish to have their relative's body donated for research if it is not suitable for organ/tissue donation. Sometimes, as in the case of patients with cancer, middle ears may be suitable for donation. The patient may be mistakenly considered "medically unsuitable" for donation.[2,5-9]

3. **A. Assessment.** If the patient had properly complied with the provisions of the Uniform Anatomical Gift Act of the state in which he or she was a resident, the request of the patient to be an organ donor would take precedence over the wishes of the patient's family. The gift takes effect immediately on death and is therefore binding on relatives. Thus technically the decision of an individual to donate an organ is legally binding on the family. In practical terms and as a matter of policy, however, few hospitals go against the wishes of family members if they choose not to proceed with donation. A common practice is to obtain consent for organ and tissue donation from the donor's next of kin.[1,2,4-6]

4. **A. Analysis.** The family is exhibiting an inability to cope with the tragic news of their family member's death. Although individuals react differently to a family member's death, violent and threatening behavior is not acceptable behavior. This family needs a lot of support, and a referral should be made to a member of the clergy or to a social worker.

5. **C. Intervention.** The timing of when organ/tissue donation is requested and the way a family is approached are key issues in obtaining consent for organ donation. Physicians and nurses may be reluctant to discuss organ donation with potential donor families, fearing that this will cause the families more distress. However, it has been found that organ donation may actually bring consolation to a grieving family.[10,11]

6. **B. Evaluation.** Ensuring organ viability is the primary goal in organ donor management. This is accomplished by maintaining optimal hydration, oxygenation, and hemodynamic stability.[2,4,5,10,11]

7. **B. Intervention.** One method that has been found useful for maintaining adequate fluid volume for the potential organ donor is the infusion of either normal saline or Ringer's lactate solution. With its lower sodium concentration, Ringer's lactate is preferred as the crystallized volume expander because of the high incidence of hypernatremia in the donor population. Packed red blood cells would be given only if the donor were hypovolemic as a result of blood loss. Albumin may be used to increase the circulating volume.*

8. **A. Intervention.** Dopamine is the vasopressor of choice for restoring autoregulatory control. If dopamine is ineffective, the second drug of choice is isoproterenol. The use of norepinephrine should be avoided, because it raises the body's oxygen demands and can constrict the vessels supplying major organs. Large doses of vasopressors should be avoided whenever possible to prevent vasoconstriction, which can also produce decreased organ perfusion.*

9. **A. Assessment/intervention.** The emergency department nurse has the responsibility of completing a detailed assessment of the hemodynamic status of the patient to enable recognition and prevention of complications leading to poor perfusion of potentially transplantable organs. Monitoring of the cardiac rate and rhythm, blood pressure, fluid intake, and urine output should be done on an hourly basis or more frequently if the patient's condition warrants it. Skin color and temperature, and the presence and quality of peripheral pulses are observed as an indication of tissue perfusion by the emergency nurse. The response of blood pressure and central venous pressure and/or pulmonary artery pressures to fluid challenges should be closely monitored and documented.[12,13]

10. **C. Intervention.** The legal priority of individuals from whom consent can be obtained for a patient's organ/tissue donation are (in this order): the patient's spouse, an adult son or daughter, either parent, an adult brother

*References 1, 2, 4, 5, 7, 12, 13.

or sister, a guardian, or any other person authorized or under obligation to dispose of the body.[7-9,14]

11. **C. Assessment.** Obesity in an otherwise healthy individual is not an exclusionary criterion for organ donation.[12,13]

12. **B. Analysis.** Exposure to foreign substances such as soot, a chemical, or water, which may contain debris or bacteria, increases the patient's potential to develop infection.[15]

REFERENCES

1. Darby J et al: Approach to the management of the heartbeating brain dead organ donor, *JAMA* 21:2222-2228, 1989.
2. Schroyer M: Organ and tissue donation: what emergency department nurses should know. In Kitt S, Kaiser J, editors: *Emergency nursing: a physiologic and clinical perspective,* Philadelphia, 1990, WB Saunders.
3. Prottas J, Batten H: *Attitudes and incentives in organ procurement. I. Professional attitudes toward organ procurement,* Report to the Health Care Financing Administration, 1986.
4. Goldsmith J, Montefusco C: Nursing care of the potential organ donor, *Crit Care Nurse* 5:22-29, 1989.
5. Cox J: Organ donation: the challenge of emergency nursing, *JEN* 12:199-204, 1986.
6. Simpson H: Understanding the law: organ donation, *Nurs Life* 5:24, 1985.
7. Williams L: Organ procurement: what nurses need to know, *Crit Care Q* 8:27-30, 1985.
8. Creighton H: *Law every nurse should know,* Philadelphia, 1986, WB Saunders.
9. Goldstein A, Perdew S, Pruitt S: *The nurse's legal advisor,* Philadelphia, 1989, JB Lippincott.
10. Report of the ad hoc committee of Harvard Medical School to examine the definitions of brain death, *JAMA* 205:337, 1968.
11. Minister's Task Force on Kidney Donation: *Organ donation in the eighties,* 1985, Ontario Ministry of Health.
12. Norris MK: How to manage tissue donation, *Am J Nurs* 10:1300-1302, 1989.
13. Snyder L, Peter N: How to manage organ donation, *Am J Nurs* 10:1294-1299, 1989.
14. Task Force on Organ Transplantation: *Organ transplantation: issues and recommendations: report of the Task Force on Organ Transplantation,* Washington, DC, 1986, US Department of Health and Human Services.
15. Carlson J et al: *Nursing diagnosis,* Philadelphia, 1991, WB Saunders.

ADDITIONAL READINGS

Peele A: The nurse's role in promoting the rights of donor families, *Nurs Clin North Am* 24:939-949, 1989.

Rea R et al: *Emergency nursing core curriculum,* ed 3, Philadelphia, 1987, WB Saunders.

Simmons RG, Simmons RL: *The gift of life,* New York, 1977, John Wiley & Sons.

Stuart F: Need, supply and legal issues related to organ transplantation in the U.S., *Transplant Proc* 16:88, 1984.

Younger et al: Brain death and organ retrieval: a cross sectional survey of knowledge and concepts among health professionals, *JAMA* 21:2205-2210, 1989.

Chapter 12

Orthopedic Emergencies

REVIEW OUTLINE

I. Anatomy and physiology
   A. Bones
   B. Major skeletal muscles
   C. Range of motion
   D. Neurovascular status affected by orthopedic injuries
      1. Circulation
      2. Sensory perception
      3. Motor function

II. Orthopedic assessment
   A. History
      1. Chief complaint
         a. Mechanism of injury
         b. Position of limb when injured
         c. Ability to use body part since injury
         d. Time of injury or onset
         e. Swelling, deformity
         f. First aid or treatment since onset
         g. Associated injuries
      2. Significant medical status
         a. Previous injury to same site
         b. Current medications
         c. Allergies
         d. Immunization status
         e. Chronic diseases
   B. Physical examination
      1. Overview
         a. Positioning

        b. Degree of distress

        c. Skin color, moisture, temperature

        d. Vital signs

     2. Affected part

        a. Deformity

        b. Swelling

        c. Ecchymosis

        d. Loss of function

        e. Abnormal position or mobility

        f. Point tenderness

        g. Lack of skin integrity

        h. 5 Ps

           (1) Pain

           (2) Pulse

           (3) Paresthesia

           (4) Paralysis

           (5) Pallor

        i. Range of motion

   C. Diagnostic studies or procedures

     1. Skeletal x-ray studies

     2. Tomography

     3. Scanning

     4. Magnetic resonance imaging

     5. Complete blood cell count (CBC) with differential

     6. Uric acid level

     7. Compartment pressure measurement

III. Related nursing diagnoses

   A. Activity intolerance

   B. Anxiety

   C. Body image disturbance

   D. Fear

   E. Fluid volume deficit (actual or potential)

   F. Infection, potential for

   G. Injury, potential for

   H. Knowledge deficit

   I. Mobility, impaired physical

   J. Pain

   K. Posttrauma response

   L. Powerlessness

   M. Self-care deficit

    N. Skin integrity, impaired (actual or potential)

    O. Tissue perfusion, altered (peripheral)

IV. Collaborative care of the patient with an orthopedic emergency

    A. Airway maintenance

    B. Bleeding/hemorrhage control

    C. Blood and fluid replacement

    D. Cardiac status monitoring

    E. Amputated part preservation

    F. Pharmacological interventions

       1. Analgesics

       2. Antibiotics

       3. Antiinflammatories

          a. Steroidal

          b. Nonsteroidal

       4. Muscle relaxants

       5. Local/regional anesthesia

    G. Immobilization

       1. Splinting

       2. Casting

       3. Traction

          a. Skin

          b. Skeletal

       4. Serial reassessment

       5. Local comfort measures

       6. Wound care

       7. Compartment pressure monitoring

       8. Emotional support

       9. Patient/family teaching

V. Specific orthopedic emergencies

    A. Sprains, strains

    B. Fractures

    C. Dislocations, subluxations

    D. Inflammatory conditions

       1. Bursitis

       2. Tendonitis

       3. Joint effusion

    E. Carpal tunnel syndrome

    F. Amputations

    G. Complications

       1. Bundle injury

2. Compartment syndrome
3. Fat embolus

INTRODUCTION

Orthopedic emergencies are responsible for a considerable number of patient visits to emergency departments. Most are related to recent injuries incurred in our fast-moving society. Motor vehicles, bicycles, falls, industrial equipment, and sports activities are all contributors to bone, joint, tendon, and muscle problems.

The musculoskeletal system is made up of 206 bones and skeletal muscle equaling 40% to 50% of body weight.[1] It has two major functions, the first of which is to provide a framework for the body. In doing so, the musculoskeletal system serves as a means of support and protection for the vital organs. The second purpose is to provide for leverage and movement of the various body parts and for the body as a whole. In considering the anatomy and physiology of this system, it is important to note that veins, arteries, and nerves follow the course of long bones and that damage to the bone may include and/or cause injury to any of these structures.

The most important nursing measure in the initial phase of caring for the patient who has an orthopedic emergency is to immediately assess the whole patient. Compound fractures, dislocations, and severe deformities have a dramatic appearance but are not life threatening. Stabilization of the ABCs (airway, breathing, circulation) is essential and should not be overlooked or delayed. An important axiom to remember is that the most obvious may not be the most severe.

In obtaining a history of the chief complaint, careful scrutiny is given to the mechanism of injury. Factors such as force involved, trajectory, position of the limb when injured, time elapsed since the incident, activity or ability to use the body part since injury, and any first aid prior to seeking care all contribute to understanding the presenting problem. In addition, this information assists in discovering associated injuries of which the patient may be unaware. A history of any previous similar injury, as well as a review of current medications, use of alcohol or other drugs, and any significant past medical history, will be helpful. Special considerations of the elderly, infants, and children include the possibility of abuse and complications such as hypothermia and dehydration.

An objective assessment of the patient with an orthopedic emergency includes observing the affected area for abnormalities such as deformity, swelling, discoloration, loss of function, and abnormal position or movement.

Palpation may reveal point tenderness or crepitus. Neurovascular status distal to the site is assessed initially and serially.

Interventions appropriate to the management of the emergency orthopedic patient include stabilizing the injured part as soon as possible. Open wounds are covered with sterile saline dressings. Splinting is performed using whatever device will immobilize the part and still allow access for circulatory checks. It is important to remember to pad the splint well and to immobilize the joint above and below the injury.

Pain control is an important facet of care. Local comfort measures of ice and elevation decrease venous congestion and therefore reduce swelling, a major factor contributing to pain. In addition, pharmacological agents are indicated. Concurrent skin defects are cleansed and dressed as indicated. The potential for infection can be significant and requires administration of antibiotics.

An orthopedic emergency of life-threatening proportion is a fractured pelvis. Significant pelvic fractures are incurred in incidents involving severe, direct force. Tears in pelvic and lumbar vessels can result in rapid, massive blood loss. With pelvic fractures it is common to have injuries in other systems as well, especially the genitourinary and gastrointestinal systems. Interventions in this instance include aggressive fluid resuscitation, application of the pneumatic antishock garment (PASG) for stabilization and tamponade effect, and rapid identification and management of associated injuries.

REVIEW QUESTIONS
Tendonitis

A 34-year-old woman comes to the emergency department complaining of right wrist pain of 1 week's duration that is gradually becoming worse. She has no history of direct trauma to the extremity. Vital signs are blood pressure, 116/82; pulse, 84; respiratory rate, 16; and temperature, 97.8° F.

1. Pertinent subjective assessment obtained by the nurse includes:
  0   A. Immunization status
  0   B. Activity prior to the onset of pain
  0   C. Previous injury to the same site
  0   D. Allergies

2. An examination of this patient's right arm reveals:
  0   A. Discoloration at or distal to the wrist
  0   B. Abnormal mobility
  0   C. Increased pain with motion
  0   D. Sensory deficit in the fingers

3. The appropriate nursing diagnosis on which to base care for this patient is:
   0   A. Mobility, impaired physical
   0   B. Infection, potential for
   0   C. Skin integrity, impaired, potential
   0   D. Tissue perfusion, altered (peripheral)

4. The physician prescribes ibuprofen for this patient. The nurse recognizes this drug as a:
   0   A. Synthetic narcotic
   0   B. Salicylate
   0   C. Tricyclic antidepressant
   0   D. Nonsteroidal antiinflammatory agent

5. In discharging this patient, the nurse instructs her to be rechecked by her physician in 1 week if she is no better. What specific instructions should the nurse give this patient for taking her medication?
   0   A. Take medication before meals
   0   B. Take medication with food or milk
   0   C. Double the dose if the medication is not effective
   0   D. Evenly space doses over a 24-hour period

Injury

A 32-year-old man is brought to the emergency department by the rescue squad after an automobile head-on collision. He was a restrained front seat passenger who required some extrication. He arrives on a long backboard awake, alert, and complaining of pain in both legs. He has some minor abrasions of the face; the left knee has a deep laceration with crepitus; and the right ankle is obviously deformed. Vital signs are blood pressure, 122/72; pulse, 106; respiratory rate, 24; and temperature, 98.4° F.

6. The nurse's first action in receiving this patient should be to:
   0   A. Immobilize the cervical spine with a Philadelphia collar
   0   B. Apply a splint to the right ankle
   0   C. Assess ABCs
   0   D. Inquire if others injured in the accident will be brought to this facility

7. While performing an objective assessment, the nurse notes that pulses are absent in the right foot. An appropriate intervention for this problem would be to:
   0   A. Splint the extremity so that no further harm may be done
   0   B. Expedite portable films of the right lower extremity

0   C. Attempt to straighten the deformity
0   D. Notify the physician at once

8. The appropriate initial x-ray films to be obtained on this patient are:
   0   A. Cross table cervical spine, chest, pelvis
   0   B. Cross table cervical spine, pelvis, left knee
   0   C. Chest, pelvis, right ankle
   0   D. Pelvis, left knee, right ankle

9. The mechanism of injury and presence of left knee injury alert the nurse to what possible associated injury?
   0   A. Left hip and/or acetabular injury
   0   B. Lumbar spine injury
   0   C. Left os calcis fracture
   0   D. Chest injury

10. The physician orders cefazolin, 1 g, and gentamycin, 160 mg IV. Which nursing diagnosis is reflected in this order?
    0   A. Pain
    0   B. Infection, potential for
    0   C. Tissue perfusion, altered (peripheral)
    0   D. Anxiety

Fat Embolus

A 26-year-old man is brought to the emergency department by the rescue squad. He is complaining of a sudden onset of shortness of breath, and he is restless and somewhat cyanotic. Vital signs are blood pressure, 102/60; pulse, 138; respiratory rate, 44; and temperature, 100.8° F.

11. The nurse's first intervention in caring for this patient is to:
    0   A. Start high-flow oxygen by means of a nonrebreathing mask
    0   B. Draw arterial blood gases
    0   C. Attach a cardiac monitor
    0   D. Establish an IV access

12. Further assessment reveals that the patient sustained fractures of his right tibia and fibula 2 days earlier in a soccer game. He was hospitalized until this morning and then discharged with a long leg cast in place. The nurse recognizes that this puts the patient at risk for:
    0   A. Embolus secondary to deep venous thrombosis
    0   B. Adult respiratory distress syndrome

0   C. Air embolus

0   D. Fat embolus

13. The initial blood gases on this patient reveal a pH of 7.21, PCO_2 of 66, PO_2 of 60, and bicarbonate level of 26. The nurse recognizes these values as:

0   A. Respiratory alkalosis

0   B. Metabolic acidosis

0   C. Respiratory acidosis

0   D. Metabolic alkalosis

14. Based on the initial evaluation, the most appropriate nursing diagnosis is:

0   A. Airway clearance, ineffective

0   B. Cardiac output, decreased

0   C. Anxiety

0   D. Gas exchange, impaired

15. The physician orders a heparin infusion. He orders 25,000 units of heparin in 500 ml of dextrose 5% in water (D_5W) to infuse at the rate of 1000 units/hr. The flow rate in milliliters per hour is:

0   A. 12

0   B. 24

0   C. 20

0   D. 6

Compartment Syndrome

A 17-year-old youth comes to the emergency department complaining of left leg pain after being struck by an automobile and pinned against a wall. His lower left leg is deformed and markedly contused. He has no other apparent injury. Vital signs are blood pressure, 128/86; pulse, 98; respiratory rate, 20; and temperature, 98.4° F.

16. The nature of this patient's injury alerts the nurse to the possibility of his developing:

0   A. Osteomyelitis

0   B. Deep venous thrombosis

0   C. Compartment syndrome

0   D. Secondary skin infection

17. Nursing assessment of this patient's lower leg includes:

0   A. Observation for skin discontinuity

0   B. Palpation of the posterior popliteal pulse
0   C. Palpation of the dorsalis pedis and posterior tibial pulses
0   D. Check for movement, sensation, and capillary refill of the toes

18. This patient is given meperidine, 50 mg IV, for pain, and a long leg splint is applied. Thirty minutes after medication administration, he continues to complain of severe pain in his left leg, which increases with movement of his toes. Sensation and capillary refill remain intact. An appropriate nursing intervention at this time would be to:
0   A. Notify the physician immediately
0   B. Adjust the splint
0   C. Reposition the leg on pillows
0   D. Administer one half the first meperidine dose

19. Measurement of compartment pressures is accomplished using a(n):
0   A. Pulse oximeter
0   B. Manometer
0   C. Sphygmomanometer
0   D. Air splint

20. Evidence of compartment syndrome may be reflected in which other system?
0   A. Pulmonary
0   B. Cardiac
0   C. Renal
0   D. Gastrointestinal

21. The nursing diagnosis that best reflects the problems of compartment syndrome is:
0   A. Pain (acute)
0   B. Gas exchange, impaired
0   C. Skin integrity, impaired, potential
0   D. Tissue perfusion, altered, peripheral

ANSWERS

1. **B. Assessment.** The most beneficial information concerning this patient's problem can be derived from learning what the patient was doing before the pain began. Most often the nurse will discover some repetitive activity involving the affected joint, in this case, the wrist.

2. **C. Assessment.** Excessive, continued stress on an area produces inflammation of the involved tendons. Movement exacerbates the pain. Frequently crepitus is also felt over the affected tendon.

3. **A. Analysis.** The goal in treatment of tendonitis is to reduce irritation by immobilizing the affected area. In addition, local application of heat may be beneficial.[1]

4. **D. Intervention.** Ibuprofen and the other nonsteroidal antiinflammatories are first-line agents for inflammatory conditions such as tendonitis. The action of these drugs is related to inhibition of prostaglandin synthesis; however, the exact method of action is not known.[2]

5. **B. Intervention.** A common side effect of the nonsteroidal antiinflammatories is gastrointestinal upset. Taking the medication with food or milk helps protect the stomach from irritation.

6. **C. Intervention.** Evaluating the status of airway, breathing, and circulation should be the automatic first response to every patient. The appearance of deformed limbs should never divert the nurse from a basic primary assessment.

7. **D. Intervention.** Initial and serial reevaluation of circulation distal to the injury is a nursing responsibility. A pulseless extremity is a serious emergency and is brought to the physician's attention at once.

8. **A. Intervention.** Initial x-ray films are taken on a patient with multiple trauma immediately after stabilizing the ABCs to rule out life-threatening injuries. A cross table cervical spine film helps identify serious neck injury. A chest film is taken to look for pneumothorax or hemothorax and for any mediastinal shift. A pelvis film will reveal fractures that could cause massive blood loss. These x-ray studies can be done quickly by portable machine and create minimal disruption of patient care.

9. **A. Assessment.** In a front-end collision the patient sustains a blow to the knee while in the flexed position. This energy is transmitted up the femur to the flexed hip joint, causing hip fracture, acetabular fracture, or posterior hip dislocation. Careful evaluation of this patient's left hip and pelvis is indicated.

10. **B. Analysis.** Compound fractures, such as this patient's left knee injury, are prime targets for serious infection. Vigorous prevention of this complication is begun early in the patient's stay.

11. **A. Intervention.** All of the interventions listed are indicated in the early care of this patient; however, the first priority is to provide supplemental oxygen. Tachypnea, restlessness, and cyanosis are clear-cut signs of respiratory distress and must be addressed immediately.

12. **D. Assessment.** A serious complication in patients who have sustained

long bone fractures is fat embolus. This phenomenon is characteristically seen 2 to 3 days after injury in the patient who is in the second or third decade. The embolization is thought to be a result of fat and marrow break-off directly related to the fracture, as well as a result of changes in circulating lipids secondary to stress.[3]

13. **C. Assessment.** Interpretation of the ABGs should begin with the pH. Normal pH is 7.35 to 7.45. Because this patient's pH is reported at 7.21, he is in a state of acidosis. Next, note the P_{CO_2}. This reflects the respiratory side of the acid-base equation. Normally the value should be 35 to 45 mm Hg. A value of 66 indicates retained carbon dioxide. A normal bicarbonate level is 22 to 26 mEq and represents the metabolic or buffer system component. The patient's value of 26 falls within the normal range. This patient's blood gases demonstrate a respiratory acidosis.[4]

14. **D. Analysis.** The respiratory compromise this patient is experiencing is at the alveolar-capillary level, where carbon dioxide–oxygen exchange occurs. Because emboli have obstructed vessels in the lungs, there is a decreased area in which gas exchange can take place.[5]

15. **C. Intervention.** 25,000 units in 500 ml is 50 units/ml. To determine the number of milliliters per hour, divide what is desired (1000 units) by what you have (50 units) to arrive at the correct amount of 20 ml/hr.

16. **C. Assessment.** Compartment syndrome is a real possibility in orthopedic injuries whose mechanism of injury is a crushing force. The most common site of development is the anterior compartment of the lower leg.[5]

17. **D. Assessment.** Compartment syndrome develops when tissue pressures within a limited space, the muscle compartment, exceed the intraarterial hydrostatic pressure, causing collapse of capillaries and venules, and subsequent tissue necrosis. Loss of a pulse distal to the affected area is a late sign. Initial and frequent checks for motion, sensation, and capillary refill are most valuable in detecting this complication early.

18. **A. Intervention.** Hallmark signs of developing compartment syndrome are severe pain not relieved by narcotics that increases with muscle stretching. This finding needs to be reported immediately, so that proper medical intervention may ensue.

19. **B. Intervention.** The quick and easy way of obtaining compartment pressures is with a setup using a three-way stopcock, IV tubing, a syringe of saline, and a mercury manometer. Normal compartment pressures should be less than 20 mm Hg.[5]

20. **C. Evaluation.** When this complication advances to the stage of muscle death, myoglobinuria and subsequent renal complications may develop.[4]

21. **D. Analysis.** This diagnosis is defined as a decrease in oxygenation and

nutrition at the cellular level due to a deficit in capillary blood supply.[6] This is an accurate physiological description of what happens in compartment syndrome.

REFERENCES

1. Tintinalli J: *Emergency medicine,* New York, 1988, McGraw-Hill.
2. Karch A, Boyd E: *Handbook of drugs,* Philadelphia, 1989, JB Lippincott.
3. Rockwood C, Green D: *Fractures in adults,* Philadelphia, 1984, JB Lippincott.
4. Sheehy SB: *Mosby's manual of emergency care,* ed 3, St Louis, 1990, Mosby–Year Book.
5. Proehl J: Compartment syndrome, *JEN* 14(5):283-290, 1988.
6. Kim MJ, McFarland GK, McLane AM: *Pocket guide to nursing diagnosis,* ed 4, St Louis, 1990, Mosby–Year Book.

ADDITIONAL READING

Rea R et al: *Emergency nursing core curriculum,* ed 3, Philadelphia, 1987, WB Saunders.

Chapter 13
Psychiatric Emergencies

REVIEW OUTLINE

I. Definition
   A. Psychiatric emergency
   B. Psychiatric crisis

II. Assessment
   A. History
      1. Chief complaint
      2. Events causing the patient to seek emergency care
      3. Past medical and/or psychiatric history
      4. Medications
      5. Allergies
   B. Physical examination
      1. Primary survey and stabilization
      2. Secondary assessment
   C. Mental status examination
      1. Behavior and general appearance
      2. Speech
      3. Mood and affect
      4. Thought processes or mental content
      5. Perception
      6. Judgment
      7. Cognitive ability
         a. Attention and concentration
         b. Basic knowledge
         c. Abstract reasoning
         d. Orientation
         e. Memory
   D. Diagnostic studies or procedures

       1. ECG
       2. Laboratory
       3. Radiology
III. Related nursing diagnoses
   A. Anxiety
   B. Communication, impaired verbal
   C. Coping, ineffective
   D. Fear
   E. Grieving, anticipatory
   F. Grieving, dysfunctional
   G. Injury (trauma), potential for
   H. Posttrauma response
   I. Powerlessness
   J. Sleep pattern disturbance
   K. Thought processes, altered
   L. Violence, potential for: self-directed or directed at others
IV. Collaborative care of the patient with a psychiatric emergency
   A. Physical care
      1. ABCDE (airway, breathing, circulation, deficit [neurological], exposure)
      2. Provide for physical safety of self, the patient, the patient's significant others, other patients, and the staff
        a. Privacy
        b. Restraints
      3. Diagnostic data
      4. Medications
   B. Emotional support
      1. Assess the patient's level of potential for violence
      2. Allow the patient to ventilate
      3. Set limits
      4. Medications
   C. Patient teaching for patient and significant other

INTRODUCTION

Violence has become a part of the American culture. Like many other features of our culture, violence has worked its way into each emergency department across our country. Not only do we as emergency nurses provide care for both victims and assailants, but all too frequently we must deal with violence as it occurs before our eyes.

To handle violence successfully, the emergency nurse must assess the patient for life-threatening illness or injury and intervene to stabilize the patient's physical condition. The emergency nurse must also assess the patient who has the potential to act violently and intervene to protect himself or herself, the patient, the patient's significant others, and other emergency department staff and patients.

Violence has many underlying causes. Some of the more common disorders associated with violence are listed in Box 1.

Violence can be directed toward the self (suicide) or others (assault, homicide). Each type has distinct signs and symptoms that must be recognized for successful treatment.

Box 1   Disorders associated with violence

Organic Disorders
Drugs
Alcohol (intoxication, withdrawal, chronic brain syndrome)
Amphetamines
Cocaine
Sedative-hypnotic intoxication or withdrawal
PCP
LSD
Anticholinergics (TCAs, neuroleptics, atropine and its derivative, OTC sedatives, and cold preparations)

Diseases
Hypoglycemia
Hypoxia
Meningitis
Head trauma
Temporal lobe epilepsy
AIDS (primary or seconday infection)
Electrolyte imbalance
Hypothermia or hyperthermia
Anemia
Dementia

Vitamin deficiencies
Endocrinopathies
Essential organ disease

Psychiatric Disorders
Mania
Schizophrenia
Paranoid states
Borderline personality

Situational Frustration
Mutual hostility
Miscommunication with staff
Fear of dependency on or rejection by staff or family
Fear of illness
Guilt over perceived role in the disease process
Long waiting time in the emergency department
Unpleasant waiting environment (insufficient, uncomfortable seating; lack of distraction, such as TV or magazines; lack of access to refreshment

Antisocial Behavior
Violence not due to medical or psychiatric causes

From Williams D, Dwyer D, editors: *Rep Emerg Nurs*, preview issue, pp 1-8, 1990.

Suicide is violence directed toward the self. The actual suicide attempt may be accomplished in a variety of ways; ingestion or inhalation of substances and self-inflicted gunshot wounds are but a few of the most common methods used. The priority of care for the patient who has attempted suicide is assessment and stabilization of life-threatening injuries (ABCDE). The secondary assessment usually begins with the history, which is very important for this particular patient. Throughout history taking, the emergency nurse tries to identify pertinent risk factors, as well as elicit information to assess the lethality or severity of the suicide attempt.

Factors associated with the lethality or severity of a suicide plan or attempt are identified in Box 2.

Interventions for the patient who has attempted suicide include the following: provide a safe environment, including physical and/or chemical restraints; allow the patient to ventilate; assist with the psychiatric consultation; and arrange for discharge home or admission to an appropriate facility.

The patient who has the potential to direct violence toward others can be easily identified, since violence rarely strikes without warning. On history taking, the nurse may find that the patient has a past medical history of homicidal or violent behavior, suicidal thoughts, psychosis, and/or substance abuse. The patient may also have a history of being abused as a child, enuresis, and/or problem behavior during childhood (fire setting, cruelty to animals,

---

Box 2   Factors associated with the lethality or severity of a suicide plan or attempt

Details of suicide plan or attempt carefully thought out over time
Believes or believed plan or attempt could or would be successful
Precautions considered or taken to avoid interruption
Precautions considered or taken to avoid discovery
Final arrangements planned or completed (e.g., purchasing life insurance, writing suicide notes, note saying goodbye to significant others)
Means of carrying out suicide plan available
Plan or method leaves little or no opportunity for survival or reversal
Wish to die is strong or wish to live is minimal or absent
In addition to the foregoing, other indications of ongoing suicide risk in persons who have already attempted suicide include:
    Suicide attempt did not accomplish what it was intended to (e.g., death, reaction from significant others)
    Patient expresses regret at being discovered or recovered

From Kitt S, Kaiser J, editors: *Emergency nursing: a physiologic and clinical perspective,* Philadelphia, 1990, WB Saunders.

fighting, school problems). A past history of head injury or organic diseases (see Box 1) may also exist.

Signs and symptoms of potential violence include:

- Provocative behavior toward the nurse or any other team member
- An angry demeanor
- Manic states
- Drunkenness or other substance use
- Delirium or confusion
- Motor restlessness
- Loud, angry, forceful speech
- Agitated behavior
- Threats to kill or injure someone
- The presence of weapons
- The nurse's "gut feeling"

The appropriate approach to the violent patient is depicted in Box 3.

One of the nursing interventions for the patient with the potential for violence includes the use of physical or chemical restraints, which should be carried out in accordance with the institution's policies and procedures. Referral to an appropriate facility for definitive care may also be necessary.

Box 3   Approach to the violent patient

1. Never see a dangerous patient alone. You should always feel completely safe when evaluating a patient. Never jeopardize your safety.
2. Do not see a patient who is carrying a weapon. Ask about weapons and have the patient empty his or her pockets, wallet, or handbag. A patient who refuses must be searched.
3. Do not touch the patient, approach too rapidly, or stand too close. Hostile persons require increased personal space, and violation of this space is perceived as an attack.
4. Keep the door open and allow unobstructed access to the door for both yourself and the patient. Both parties should feel that they can leave the room immediately if the situation becomes dangerous.
5. Do not sit behind a desk, have your arms or legs tangled up as you sit, or otherwise compromise your ability to get away from the patient.
6. Do not argue with or challenge the patient's self-esteem. Rather, emphasize how much strength it takes to remain calm and cooperative.
7. Call the police if the patient becomes too threatening.
8. Never attempt to subdue the patient alone or otherwise be a hero.

From Williams D, Dwyer D, editors: *Rep Emerg Nurse,* preview issue, pp 1-8, 1990.

REVIEW QUESTIONS

Suicide

Jane, a 16-year-old teenager, is brought to the emergency department by the rescue squad for treatment of superficial lacerations to her wrist. She is crying and states that she hates her mother for making her come to the hospital. Jane states that she cut herself because her boyfriend broke up with her. She is awake, alert, and oriented. Both Jane and her mother state that Jane has never done anything like this before.

1. The lethality of Jane's suicide attempt would be assessed as:
   - 0   A. Low
   - 0   B. High

Mr. Jay, a 23-year-old man, is brought to the emergency department by the rescue squad because of attempted suicide. Mr. Jay had reportedly locked himself in the garage and started his car, attempting suicide by carbon monoxide poisoning. Mr. Jay's mother arrived home unexpectedly early, discovered him, opened the garage door, and called the rescue squad. On arrival in the emergency department, Mr. Jay is intubated and agitated. The paramedics report that he was unresponsive at the scene with stable vital signs and was intubated for airway protection only. Mr. Jay's mother explains that he has been depressed for several years since his father died of cancer. He has made previous suicide attempts. Mr. Jay's mother also states that she found a suicide note on the kitchen table.

2. The lethality of Mr. Jay's suicide attempt would be assessed as:
   - 0   A. Low
   - 0   B. High

3. The first priority of care for Mr. Jay would be to:
   - 0   A. Assess the airway for placement of the endotracheal tube
   - 0   B. Assess vital signs
   - 0   C. Start an IV infusion and give diazepam
   - 0   D. Call the chaplain to sit with Mr. Jay's mother

4. An appropriate nursing diagnosis for Mr. Jay would be:
   - 0   A. Anxiety
   - 0   B. Posttrauma response
   - 0   C. Thought processes, altered
   - 0   D. Violence (actual): self-directed

5. Mr. Jay's airway is patent, and oxygen saturation is adequate. His vital signs are stable. Mr. Jay's agitation continues. Diazepam, 5 mg IV, is ordered. The nurse is aware of the potential side effects of this drug and monitors Mr. Jay's:
   0   A. Respirations
   0   B. Pulse
   0   C. Bowel sounds
   0   D. Pupils

Violent Behavior

Mr. White, a 24-year-old man, comes to the triage desk, pounds his fist on the desk, and states, "I need to see a doctor now!" There is an odor of alcohol on his breath. He has several abrasions on his face, and his clothing is soiled and torn. When the nurse asks Mr. White what happened, he replies, "It's none of your *#?/ business!"

6. Mr. White's potential for violence would be assessed as:
   0   A. High
   0   B. Low

7. The initial nursing intervention should be to:
   0   A. Tell Mr. White to shut up and sit down
   0   B. Take Mr. White immediately into the emergency department
   0   C. Ask Mr. White to please wait, while removing oneself from the situation and calling for help
   0   D. Take Mr. White's hand, tell him it is apparent that he is upset, and ask him if he wants to talk about his anger

Ms. Brown, a 32-year-old woman, comes to the emergency department as a victim of spousal abuse. She has an obvious deformity of the nose but no other injuries. She is awake, oriented, and crying. Her vital signs are stable. It is an extremely busy day, and Ms. Brown may need to wait to be seen.

8. Ms. Brown's potential for violent behavior would be assessed as:
   0   A. High
   0   B. Low

9. Ms. Brown begins to pace and continues to cry. An appropriate verbal intervention would be:

    0   A. "It looks like you are feeling restless. Can you tell me what is making you nervous?"

    0   B. "I know you've been waiting to be seen, but we're very busy with more serious problems."

    0   C. "Please stop pacing. You're making everyone here nervous."

    0   D. "If you don't stop pacing, your nose may start to bleed."

10. An appropriate nursing diagnosis for Ms. Brown would be:
- 0 A. Airway clearance, ineffective
- 0 B. Breathing pattern, ineffective
- 0 C. Rape-trauma syndrome
- 0 D. Anxiety

Organic Disease

Mr. Johnson, a 66-year-old man, is brought to the emergency department by the rescue squad because of uncontrollable behavior. Mr. Johnson reportedly boarded a bus and began yelling at the other passengers. The police were called when Mr. Johnson refused to leave the bus. Mr. Johnson is restrained. He answers all questions by screaming, "Let me go!"

11. The initial nursing intervention should be to:
- 0 A. Assess the airway for patency
- 0 B. Move Mr. Johnson from the squad to the emergency department stretcher and maintain restraints
- 0 C. Start an IV infusion and give diazepam
- 0 D. Let Mr. Johnson go

12. Additional nursing intervention(s) would be to:
- 0 A. Check the patient's blood glucose level by finger stick
- 0 B. Check the patient's oxygen saturation by pulse oximetry
- 0 C. Check the patient's pupils
- 0 D. All of the above

13. An appropriate nursing diagnosis for Mr. Johnson would be:
- 0 A. Role performance, altered
- 0 B. Violence, potential for: directed at others
- 0 C. Health maintenance, altered
- 0 D. Personal identity disturbance

14. Mr. Johnson is found to be hypoglycemic. An IV infusion is started, and dextrose is given by IV push. Mr. Johnson calms down and starts asking, "Where am I?" The nurse explains to Mr. Johnson what has happened, and he becomes embarrassed. Is it appropriate to remove Mr. Johnson's restraints at this time?

0   A. Yes
0   B. No

15. Mr. Johnson reveals that he is a diabetic. He took his insulin this morning, but did not eat. He is given a sandwich and orange juice. Mr. Johnson should be observed for:

0   A. Hyperglycemia
0   B. Hypoglycemia
0   C. Elevated intracranial pressure
0   D. Self-destructive behavior

ANSWERS

1. **A. Assessment.** Jane's suicide attempt ranks low in lethality because of her age and sex. This is also her first attempt at suicide, and the attempt was not well planned.
2. **B. Assessment.** Mr. Jay's suicide attempt ranks high in lethality because of his age, sex, history of depression, and previous attempts. Mr. Jay's plan was well thought out and unsuccessful only because his mother arrived home unexpectedly early. He had also written a suicide note.
3. **A. Intervention.** The ABCs remain the priority of nursing care for Mr. Jay. The endotracheal tube should be assessed for patency after each patient transfer (from squad stretcher to emergency department bed). It also needs to be assessed for patency, since Mr. Jay was previously unresponsive but is now agitated. The paramedics report that Mr. Jay's vital signs were stable at the scene and that he was intubated for protection of the airway only. Restlessness is a sign of hypoxia.
4. **D. Analysis.** Answers *A, B,* and *C* can only be evaluated in the awake patient.
5. **A. Evaluation.** Diazepam is a respiratory depressant. It is particularly important to monitor Mr. Jay's respirations, since carbon monoxide poisoning is treated by oxygen administration. Carbon monoxide is also eliminated from the body by the lungs. Any decrease in respirations will inhibit successful treatment.
6. **A. Assessment.** Mr. White is exhibiting several signs of potentially violent behavior. He is pounding his fist on the desk, speaking loudly, and cursing; he has alcohol on his breath; and he appears to have been involved in a fight. The likelihood of his striking out is very high.

7. **C. Intervention.** Answer *A* would only further irritate Mr. White. Answer *B* would jeopardize the safety of other staff and patients. Answer *D* would also irritate Mr. White; one should never touch an angry patient. Answer *C* is correct because the nurse's first priority should be his or her own physical safety; thus removing oneself and calling for help is correct.

8. **A. Assessment.** Ms. Brown is very likely to become violent. She is the victim of spousal abuse, which is a situation wherein the victim may feel guilty about her (or his) own involvement in the situation. She is crying, and will have to wait to be seen. All are positive indications for violent behavior.

9. **A. Intervention.** Identifying her behavior and asking her in a nonthreatening way if she wishes to ventilate her feelings would be the appropriate way to address Ms. Brown at this time.

10. **D. Analysis.** Anxiety is the appropriate nursing diagnosis for Ms. Brown at this time. None of the other selections is appropriate.

11. **B. Intervention.** It is important to maintain restraints on the patient at this time to provide for the safety of the patient, as well as the staff. Assessment of airway patency can be quickly done when the patient screams, "Let me go!"

12. **D. Intervention.** All of the selections are appropriate answers, since it is important to rule out a physical reason for Mr. Johnson's behavior. The underlying cause of violent or aberrant behavior should be identified, if possible, and treated.

13. **B. Analysis.** The appropriate nursing diagnosis at this time should address Mr. Johnson's potential for violence.

14. **A. Intervention.** The cause of Mr. Johnson's behavior has been identified and treated. His mental status has improved. He is cooperative and should be unrestrained at this time.

15. **B. Evaluation.** Mr. Johnson should be observed for a recurrent bout of hypoglycemia.

ADDITIONAL READINGS

Cousins A: Assessment of childhood and adolescent depression and suicide potential, *JEN* 12(1):35-37, 1986.

Kitt S, Kaiser J, editors: *Emergency nursing: a physiologic and clinical perspective,* Philadelphia, 1990, WB Saunders.

Kurlowicz L: Violence in the emergency department, *Am J Nurs* 90(9):35-39, 1990.

Rea R et al: *Emergency nursing core curriculum,* ed 3, Philadelphia, 1987, WB Saunders.

Williams D, Dwyer D, editors: Safe strategies for recognizing and managing violent patients, *Rep Emerg Nurs,* preview issue, pp 1-8, 1990.

Chapter 14

Psychological Emergencies

REVIEW OUTLINE

I. Sudden death (loss) and grief
  A. The concept of loss
    1. Anticipatory grieving
    2. Loss of bodily functions
    3. Loss of a family member or loved one
    4. Loss of belongings (e.g., house in a fire)
    5. Loss of self-esteem (e.g., sexual assault, child or elderly abuse)
  B. Grief process
    1. Informing the patient or family
    2. Anger
    3. Reacting to the loss (e.g., crying, screaming, throwing things)
    4. Acceptance and coping skills
    5. Return to activities
II. Sudden infant death[1]
  A. Children at risk
    1. Major cause of death in children under the age of 1 year
    2. History of sudden infant death syndrome (SIDS) in the family
    3. Social and psychological family environment
    4. Parental stress
    5. History of child abuse
  B. Other causes of death
    1. Cardiac abnormalities
    2. Seizures
    3. Infections
    4. Metabolic abnormalities
    5. Toxins

6. Immunizations
7. Child abuse
8. Anatomical abnormalities
   C. Nursing interventions
1. Obtaining a history of the incident
2. Identification of risk factors
3. Identification of support resources for the parents and emergency department staff
III. Human abuse
   A. Child abuse
1. Identification of children at risk
2. Identification of patterns of injury
3. History related to the injury from both the parent and the child
4. Notification of appropriate authorities
   B. Elderly abuse
1. Identification of elderly adults at risk
2. Identification of patterns of injury
3. History related to the injury from both the elderly adult and the caregiver
4. Notification of appropriate authorities
5. Referral for support systems
   C. Sexual assault
1. Identification of patterns of injury
2. Documentation of injuries
3. Documentation of the history of the incident
4. Collection and preservation of the evidence
5. Treatment of potential venereal diseases
6. Follow-up care: crisis intervention for the victim and family
7. Postcoital contraception
IV. Nursing interventions for psychological emergencies
   A. Initial assessment and stabilization of the ABCs (airway, breathing, circulation)
   B. Identification of the pattern(s) of injury
   C. History of the incident from both the victim and the caregiver
   D. Notification of appropriate authorities and/or social agencies
   E. Collection and preservation of evidence
   F. Allowing the family to see the patient before death if possible
   G. Allowing the family to view the body after death
   H. Keeping the family informed during the resuscitation process
   I. Providing the family with information about death preparation

    J. Allowing the family privacy
    K. Knowledge about religious beliefs
    L. Knowledge about death customs
    M. Supportive crisis intervention with the family
V. Related nursing diagnoses
    A. Anxiety
    B. Coping, ineffective family
    C. Coping, ineffective individual
    D. Fear
    E. Grieving, anticipatory
    F. Grieving, dysfunctional
    G. Injury, potential for
    H. Pain
    I. Parenting, altered
    J. Rape-trauma syndrome
    K. Spiritual distress (distress of the human spirit)

INTRODUCTION

The emergency department nurse faces a variety of psychological emergencies, including sudden death and grief, sexual assault, SIDS, and many forms of abuse, such as child and elderly abuse.

The emergency care of these patients is complex. The patient may have suffered not only psychological injuries, but physical injuries as well. In addition, since criminal prosecution may be involved, the emergency nurse is in many cases responsible for the collection and preservation of evidence. Notifying the appropriate authorities and/or social agencies is an additional nursing intervention that needs to be completed before the patient leaves the emergency department.

Since patients who encounter psychological emergencies have little time to prepare for these crises, they depend a great deal on the emergency nurse to provide them with both physical care and emotional support. The families of these patients—particularly when the patient does not survive—look to the emergency nurse for assistance in coping with the sudden loss they are asked to confront.

Even though psychological emergencies may represent a limited number of patient encounters in the emergency department, they can be very challenging and sometimes quite difficult for the emergency department nurse.

REVIEW QUESTIONS
Sudden Death and Grief

A 16-year-old boy is brought to the emergency department by the helicopter flight team after having been accidentally shot in the neck by his friend. He arrives in full cardiac arrest.

A history obtained from the flight nurse reveals that the patient was shot in his basement, was able to walk up the stairs to ask his sister for help, and then collapsed. His sister, who is an intensive care nurse, performed the initial CPR on the patient until the paramedics and flight team arrived.

After 20 minutes of additional resuscitation, the emergency physician pronounces the patient dead.

1. The emergency nursing assessment of this patient's sister should include
   - O   A. Any history of allergies
   - O   B. Insurance coverage
   - O   C. Funeral home preference
   - O   D. Whether the sister is alone

2. One of the best interventions that can be provided for the survivors of patients who suddenly die in the emergency department is:
   - O   A. Providing the family with sedation
   - O   B. Providing the family with privacy
   - O   C. Providing the patient with the name of a local funeral home
   - O   D. Telling the family that it will be "all right" in about a year

3. After being told that her brother is dead, the patient's sister begins screaming and states that she should have done more. Which of the following nursing diagnoses should the emergency nurse use to provide care for this patient's sister?
   - O   A. Powerlessness
   - O   B. Fear
   - O   C. Anxiety
   - O   D. Injury, potential for

4. One method that the emergency nurse may use to evaluate the effectiveness of the interventions used for the family who has suffered a sudden loss (as in this case) would be to:
   - O   A. Contact the family's chaplain by phone
   - O   B. Contact the family by phone
   - O   C. Read the charting that was completed during the resuscitation
   - O   D. Consult the hospital's social service department

Sudden Infant Death Syndrome

A 3-month-old male infant is brought to the emergency department by the paramedics. The child was found by his mother to be unresponsive after having been fed and put to bed. The infant is cyanotic, cold, and without any vital signs; he is pronounced dead by the emergency physician.

5. Signs and symptoms of SIDS as a cause of death include all of the following *except:*
- 0   A. Normal hydration
- 0   B. Blood-tinged emesis
- 0   C. Pooled blood in the face
- 0   D. Bruising of the chest and arms

6. A critical emergency nursing intervention for the parents of an infant who has died from SIDS would be encouraging the parents to:
- 0   A. Call a chaplain
- 0   B. Have another child as soon as possible
- 0   C. Hold and touch the infant
- 0   D. Consent to an autopsy

7. Because of the loss of a child, the emergency nurse should base the nursing care on the following nursing diagnosis:
- 0   A. Family processes, altered
- 0   B. Fear
- 0   C. Social isolation
- 0   D. Trauma, potential for

8. Audit criteria for the care plan of the family of the infant who has died of SIDS should include all of the following *except:*
- 0   A. Referral to a local SIDS group
- 0   B. A follow-up phone call from the emergency nurse
- 0   C. Giving the family additional information, such as *Facts About Sudden Infant Death* [2]
- 0   D. Teaching the family the warning signs of SIDS

Child Abuse

An 8-week-old female infant is brought to the emergency department by her parents. They state that she has been vomiting and having diarrhea for the past 24 hours. The parents also state that the child has recently fallen down the basement stairs.

The triage nurse notes that the child has only been staring and is not moving her left side. Her blood pressure is 70 by palpation, and her pulse is 180. Discoloration is noted around her right eye.

9. One of the assessment parameters the emergency nurse may use in a case such as this when child abuse is suspected is:
   0   A. Growth and development
   0   B. Laboratory values
   0   C. Immunization history
   0   D. Current medications

10. When child abuse is suspected (as in this case), the emergency nurse must:
    0   A. Notify the parents of the nurse's suspicions
    0   B. Report the abuse to the appropriate authorities
    0   C. Obtain the appropriate consent for further treatment
    0   D. Consult with an attorney

• • •

11. A 5-year-old boy, brought to the emergency department by his teacher, is complaining about his stomach hurting. Initial evaluation reveals a child who will not make eye contact with the emergency nurse, is wearing diapers, and is clinging to his teacher. Of the following, which nursing diagnosis is most appropriate?
    0   A. Health maintenance, altered
    0   B. Growth and development, altered
    0   C. Thought processes, altered
    0   D. Grieving, dysfunctional

Elderly Abuse

A 75-year-old man is sent to the emergency department from the nursing home because his urinary catheter is not functioning. The patient is unable to speak and has soft restraints on both wrists. On evaluation of the catheter, the emergency nurse finds that the catheter has left a large laceration under the surface of the patient's penis. There is a large amount of serosanguineous drainage coming from the wound.

12. The patient's condition suggests the possibility of neglect or abuse. The initial assessment of this patient should include the identification of:
    0   A. Any belligerent behavior
    0   B. Bruises and lacerations
    0   C. Blood in his stool
    0   D. Lack of exercise

13. One of the most vital emergency nursing interventions for the elderly patient who has been abused is:

0   A. Acting as a patient advocate
0   B. Listening to the patient's caregivers
0   C. Planning patient discharge
0   D. Teaching other health care professionals about elderly abuse

14. Because of the large wound from the Foley catheter, the most appropriate nursing diagnosis on which to base this patient's care is:

0   A. Incontinence, functional
0   B. Infection, potential for
0   C. Knowledge deficit
0   D. Communication, impaired verbal

15. Audit criteria for this patient (or any patient suspected of being abused) should include:

0   A. The patient's financial status
0   B. What part of town the patient lives in
0   C. Notification of the appropriate agencies
0   D. What language the patient understands

ANSWERS

1. **D. Assessment.** An individual who is facing a sudden death or loss—particularly the loss of the child—will need the support of other family members and friends. Family members and friends can help the survivor by meeting some of the safety, security, and belongingness needs.[2]

2. **B. Intervention.** Having a private place in which to grieve is important. The family's religious and cultural background will influence the family's response to the loss of their loved one, and this privacy can allow the family members to cry, scream, and openly comfort each other without "outside" interference. A recent study found that survivors of sudden death identified the need for a private room as their primary need while in the emergency department.[2,3]

3. **A. Analysis.** The nursing diagnosis of powerlessness would be appropriate for the care of this patient's sister. Defining characteristics of this nursing diagnosis include verbalization of the feeling that one has no control over the situation or the outcome of the situation; expression of doubt about one's role performance (particularly in this case, since the

sister is an intensive care nurse), and expressions of dissatisfaction and frustrations over the inability to perform previous tasks and/or activities.[4]

4. **B. Evaluation.** One of the best methods of evaluating the effectiveness of the emergency nurse's interventions during a crisis such as in this case would be to contact the patient's family. This would provide the family members an opportunity to ask any questions that they may have forgotten, as well as suggest other interventions that may be helpful.[3]

5. **D. Assessment.** Normal hydration, blood-tinged emesis, and pooling of blood in the face and buttocks are symptoms that may accompany SIDS. However, bruising of the chest and arms could be a sign of abuse. It is important for the emergency nurse to obtain a detailed history of the circumstances surrounding the child's death to evaluate the unfortunate possibility of child abuse.[1,2]

6. **C. Intervention.** The loss of an infant from SIDS occurs with no anticipation by the infant's parents. In most cases the child was put to bed without difficulty, only to be found lifeless. It is important to encourage the parents to view the child's body, hold the child, and say good-bye. Some parents may not be able to do this, however, and the emergency nurse must be able to accept this without judging the parents.[2]

7. **A. Analysis.** Related factors contributing to this nursing diagnosis include situational transition and/or crises such as disaster, economic crisis, and change in family roles. Developmental transition and/or crises include loss of a family member, such as the infant who dies of SIDS.[4]

8. **D. Evaluation.** The care of the family whose child has died of SIDS includes referral to a local SIDS group for support, a follow-up phone call to the family to answer any questions about the infant's care in the emergency department, and the provision of any additional information that may be helpful. Since many parents tend to blame themselves for the child's death, information such as on the warning signs of SIDS would only contribute to their guilt.[2]

9. **A. Assessment.** Knowledge about growth and development can provide the emergency nurse with important information about whether this child may have been abused. In this case study, for example, the history of what supposedly happened to the child should alert the emergency nurse to the possibility of abuse: an 8-week-old infant who is not ambulatory could not have "fallen down the stairs." Signs of abuse include wounds in various stages of healing, specific patterns to injuries, injuries incompatible with the reported history of the incident, and injuries incompatible with the developmental level of the child.[2,5]

10. **B. Intervention.** In all 50 states health professionals are required to

report suspected child abuse and neglect to children's services boards, the department of public welfare, or a police officer.[5]

11. **B. Analysis.** Children can be either physically or emotionally abused. When children are consistently abused, they begin to experience changes in their growth and development.[5] The information presented in this question describes a child who is not displaying appropriate growth and development skills. The defining characteristics of this nursing diagnosis include delayed, altered, or compromised development of motor skills, adaptive skills, communication skills, and social skills.[4]

12. **B. Assessment.** From the state of the patient's catheter, it appears that the patient is already suffering the effects of neglect. The emergency nurse should assess the patient for the possibility of abuse. For the elderly patient, this should include assessment of the patient's state of hydration, nutrition, and hygiene; the patient's orientation; the presence of surface injuries; and the presence of injuries in various stages of healing.[2]

13. **A. Intervention.** The most significant emergency nursing intervention that can be provided by the emergency nurse is to act as the patient's advocate. The emergency nurse has the opportunity to identify elderly patients at risk for abuse and neglect, as well as patients who are being abused, and initiate the appropriate patient referrals.[2]

14. **B. Analysis.** The presence of the wound on the patient's penis puts him at risk for infection. Risk factors related to this nursing diagnosis include age, inadequate cellular response, unsanitary living conditions, and malnutrition.[4]

15. **C. Evaluation.** When the emergency nurse suspects that the patient may have suffered abuse, it is important that the appropriate authorities be notified. The emergency nurse may provide the patient with the only opportunity to be helped.[2]

REFERENCES

1. Goldhagen J: Infantile apnea: evaluation and management in the acute care setting. In Barkin RM, editor: *The emergently ill child*, Rockville, Md, 1987, Aspen.

2. Fought S, Throwe A: *Psychological nursing care of the emergency patient*, New York, 1987, John Wiley & Sons.

3. Fraser S, Atkins J: Survivors' recollections of helpful and unhelpful emergency nurse activities surrounding sudden death of a loved one, *JEN* 16:13-16, 1990.

4. McFarland GK, McFarlane EA: *Nursing diagnosis and intervention: planning for patient care*, St Louis, 1989, Mosby–Year Book.

5. Litwak K, Sloan M: Physical assessment of abuse, *Top Acute Care Trauma Rehabil* 2:10-16, 1987.

Chapter 15

Respiratory Emergencies

REVIEW OUTLINE

I. Anatomy and physiology
    A. Anatomy
        1. Nasal cavity
        2. Oropharynx
        3. Mucous membrane
        4. Larynx
        5. Epiglottis
        6. Vocal cords
        7. Cricothyroid membrane
        8. Trachea
        9. Bronchi
        10. Bronchioles
        11. Alveoli
        12. Lung parenchyma (right three lobes; left two lobes)
        13. Pleura
        14. Mediastinum, sternum, manubrium, xiphoid process
        15. Clavicle
        16. Ribs
        17. Thoracic vertebrae
        18. Esophagus
        19. Heart
        20. Diaphragm
        21. Intercostal muscles
        22. Accessory muscles
        23. Expiratory muscles
        24. Aorta
        25. Nerves associated with respirations

    B. Physiology
        1. Oxygen transport, gas exchange
        2. Ventilation: inspiration, expiration
        3. Tidal volume
        4. Nervous system innervation
        5. Positive-negative pressure flow system

II. Assessment
    A. Inspection
        1. Airway patency
        2. Use of accessary muscles
        3. Skin color
        4. Cyanosis
        5. Flaring of nares
        6. Sternal retraction
        7. Tachypnea
        8. Bradypnea
        9. Apnea .
      10. Splinting
      11. Audible wheezing
      12. Productive cough: sputum
    B. Palpation
        1. Pain, tenderness
        2. Crepitus
        3. Skin temperature
    C. Percussion
        1. Hollow sound
        2. Dull sound
    D. Auscultation
        1. Evaluate all lung fields
        2. Inspiration, expiration
        3. Wheezes
        4. Rhonchi
        5. Absence of breath sounds
    E. History
        1. Onset of symptoms
        2. History of trauma, mechanism of injury
        3. Pain on inspiration
        4. Cough
        5. Fever, chills
        6. Smoking history

    7. Past medical history

    8. Productive cough: sputum

    9. Work history (e.g., "black lung")

    10. Associated diseases (e.g., heart disease, emphysema, asthma, allergies)

  F. Diagnostic studies or procedures

    1. Chest x-ray studies

    2. Arterial blood gases

    3. ECG

    4. Sputum evaluation

    5. Complete blood cell count (CBC), renal, amylase, cardiac enzymes

III. Related nursing diagnoses

  A. Airway clearance, ineffective

  B. Anxiety

  C. Aspiration, potential for

  D. Breathing pattern, ineffective

  E. Fatigue

  F. Fear

  G. Gas exchange, impaired

  H. Infection, potential for

  I. Knowledge deficit

  J. Pain

IV. Collaborative care of the patient with a respiratory emergency

  A. Airway management

    1. Airway adjuncts

    2. Delivery of oxygen

    3. Intubation

  B. Ventilation

    1. Bronchodilators

    2. Humidification

  C. Cardiac monitor

  D. Antibiotics

  E. Thoracentesis

  F. Autotransfusion

  G. Chest tube insertion

  H. Thoracotomy

V. Specific respiratory emergencies

  A. Chest pain differentiation

  B. Asthma

  C. Emphysema

    D. Smoke inhalation
    E. Chronic obstructive pulmonary disease
    F. Pneumonia
    G. Adult respiratory distress syndrome (ARDS)
    H. Pulmonary embolus
    I. Hyperventilation syndrome
    J. Near-drowning
    K. Epiglottitis

INTRODUCTION

The emergency nursing assessment of the patient with respiratory distress, no matter what the cause, should include airway patency, as well as the patient's ability to keep the airway patent; the history of any specific respiratory disease and how it has been or is being treated; vital signs; auscultation of the chest; and laboratory studies, such as blood gases, a CBC, and a theophylline level when indicated. A chest x-ray film and peak expiratory flow (PEF) may also be evaluated. The amount of data that is collected in relation to the patient's respiratory distress will depend on the patient's history and the patient's ability to provide information. Many patients with chronic respiratory problems who develop distress are quite well versed in the treatment of their disease and can be a good source of information concerning what they need.

Chest Pain

The assessment of the patient with chest pain can cause some difficult problems for the emergency nurse. There are numerous causes of chest pain, including those that require emergent interventions and those that may require little if any nursing and/or medical care.

The origins of chest pain may include asthma, acute bronchitis, chronic obstructive pulmonary disease (COPD), pneumonia, pulmonary embolus, and/or a traumatic injury to the chest that may result in rib fractures, pulmonary contusion, pneumothorax, or hemothorax.

Asthma

Asthma is a response of the lung to various stimuli that cause narrowing of the airway. These stimuli may include specific allergens, such as dust and molds, stress, or intoxicants.[1,2] Even though asthma is frequently successfully treated in the emergency department, the death rate from acute asthma has been increasing.[3]

Chest Trauma

Chest trauma accounts for approximately 25% of deaths related to trauma.[4] The patient with chest trauma requires a rapid and organized emergency nursing assessment so that injuries and potential threats to life, such as a tension pneumothorax, can be rapidly identified and appropriate interventions provided.

It is important to keep in mind that trauma to the chest does not result in injury to the chest only. Contained in the thoracic cavity are the heart, great vessels, and some abdominal organs. Injuries to any of these vessels or organs can be life threatening.

Pediatric Respiratory Emergencies

The most common cause of cardiopulmonary arrest in the pediatric patient is interference with the child's airway and ventilation.[5] This can result from a disease process, such as epiglottitis, or from trauma, such as to the head or lungs.

Signs and symptoms of pediatric respiratory distress include the following: increased respiratory rate, decreased respiratory rate, apnea, fatigue, head bobbing, stridor, prolonged expiration, grunting, retractions, nasal flaring, altered mental status and cyanosis.[6,7]

REVIEW QUESTIONS
Asthma

A 30-year-old man comes to the emergency department complaining of shortness of breath. The patient states that he has been treated for asthma in the past and has not taken any medication for over a month.

1. What specific physical signs may indicate acute respiratory distress in the adult asthmatic patient?
   0   A. Paroxysmal coughing
   0   B. Sternocleidomastoid retractions
   0   C. Audible wheezing
   0   D. Vomiting

2. This patient has a PEF of less than 80 L/min. This is an indication of:
   0   A. Moderate obstruction
   0   B. No obstruction
   0   C. Severe obstruction
   0   D. Minor obstruction

3. After the ABCs (airway, breathing, circulation) of the asthmatic patient have been assessed and stabilized, what would be the next appropriate intervention?

   0   A. Administration of a corticosteroid

   0   B. Administration of theophylline

   0   C. Administration of a bronchodilator

   0   D. Administration of an antibiotic

4. An initial nursing diagnosis for the patient having an acute asthmatic attack may be:

   0   A. Health maintenance, altered

   0   B. Fluid volume excess

   0   C. Activity intolerance

   0   D. Anxiety

5. An indication that the asthmatic patient may need to be intubated would include all of the following *except:*

   0   A. A change in mental status, such as confusion, agitation, or unresponsiveness

   0   B. Respiratory arrest

   0   C. Blood gas results of pH, 7.35; PO_2, 100; and PCO_2, 40

   0   D. Inability of the patient to talk

Pneumonia

A 62-year-old woman comes to the emergency department complaining of short-ness of breath, fever, and chills. She states that she has a productive cough of yellow sputum. A chest x-ray film is obtained that shows a right lower lobe in-filtrate. The patient has a white blood cell count of 15,000. The diagnosis of pneumonia is made.

6. Pneumonia, an acute infection of the lung parenchyma, may be caused by all of the following *except:*

   0   A. Mycoplasma

   0   B. Legionella

   0   C. AIDS

   0   D. Streptococcus

7. An important nursing intervention for the patient being treated for pneumonia is:

0   A. Ordering the appropriate antibiotic
0   B. Providing the patient with fluids
0   C. Intubating the patient
0   D. Ordering a blood gas analysis

Chest Pain

A 30-year-old woman comes to the emergency department with severe chest pain, shortness of breath, and diaphoresis. Her blood pressure (palpable) is 80, her monitor shows a sinus tachycardia, and her respiratory rate is 48.

8. When obtaining a history from this patient specific to the chest pain, the emergency nurse should ask about:
   0   A. Any history of recent surgery
   0   B. The patient's last chest x-ray film
   0   C. The patient's occupation
   0   D. Any history of hyperventilation

9. Based on the patient's history of recent surgery, the emergency physician decides that the patient may be suffering from a pulmonary embolus. What medication may be started in the emergency department to treat this patient?   ·
   0   A. Heparin calcium
   0   B. Dicumarol
   0   C. Dipyridamole
   0   D. Vitamin K

10. Based on the patient's blood pressure, the following would be an appropriate nursing diagnosis:
    0   A. Injury, potential for
    0   B. Tissue perfusion, altered (cardiopulmonary)
    0   C. Thought processes, altered
    0   D. Skin integrity, impaired

11. The patient is given a bolus of 10,000 units of heparin, and a drip is begun at the rate of 1000 units/hr. Potential complications with the use of heparin include:
    0   A. Formation of clots
    0   B. Chills, fever, and urticaria
    0   C. Oral and rectal bleeding
    0   D. All of the above

Pediatric Medical Respiratory Emergencies

12. A 5-year-old girl is brought to the emergency department by her family. Her parents state that she has been febrile, lethargic, and unable to lie down; she has also been drooling. During the initial assessment of this patient, the emergency nurse should do all of the following *except:*
    0   A. Assess the child's level of consciousness
    0   B. Look down the child's throat
    0   C. Assess the child's respiratory status
    0   D. Assess the child's circulatory status

13. The initial care for the child who is suffering respiratory distress from acute epiglottitis would include:
    0   A. Administration of chloramphenicol
    0   B. Administration of racemic epinephrine
    0   C. Obtaining x-ray films of the child's neck
    0   D. Preparing the child for intubation

14. A mother comes to the emergency department carrying her 18-month-old child, who has stridor and is cyanotic. The mother states that the child was eating a hot dog before her symptoms began. The emergency nurse's initial interventions should include:
    0   A. Opening the child's mouth and trying to remove the food
    0   B. Delivering four back blows and four chest thrusts
    0   C. Grabbing the child by the legs and turning her upside down
    0   D. Performing a needle cricothyrotomy

15. The emergency nurse performs the appropriate sequence of foreign body airway obstruction (FBAO) management for the conscious infant. An indication that the maneuvers are not being effective would be:
    0   A. Expulsion of the object
    0   B. The child begins to cry
    0   C. The child becomes unconscious
    0   D. The child's color improves

16. The most common item aspirated by the child under age 3 years is:
    0   A. A toy
    0   B. A hot dog
    0   C. A peanut
    0   D. Hard candy

17. Recent evidence in the management of the child having an acute asthma attack suggests that the following intervention has been found to be very effective:

   0   A. Bronchodilation with beta-agonist
   0   B. Hydration with IV fluids
   0   C. Administration of high-flow oxygen by mask
   0   D. Administration of prophylactic antibiotics

18. A 3-month-old infant is brought to the emergency department by his parents because of a "stuffy" nose and difficulty breathing. When teaching the parents how to care for the sick infant, the emergency nurse should be sure that the parents understand all of the following *except:*

   0   A. Infants lose fluids through rapid breathing
   0   B. Infants are obligate nose breathers
   0   C. Infants cry when sick and may never be consoled
   0   D. Infants need to be kept warm but not made excessively warm

Chest Trauma

Pneumothorax

A 30-year-old man has attempted suicide by shooting himself in the left upper chest. On arrival in the emergency department, the patient is alert, is complaining of shortness of breath, and is pale and diaphoretic. His vital signs are blood pressure (palpable), 80; pulse, 140; and respiratory rate, 32.

19. The emergency nurse needs to assess quickly for the presence of:

   0   A. Breath sounds
   0   B. Peripheral edema
   0   C. Capillary refill
   0   D. Peripheral pulses

20. The emergency nurse finds that the patient does not have any breath sounds on the left side. Until a physician is available, an intervention the emergency nurse may perform in order to increase the patient's airflow is:

   0   A. Insertion of a CVP line
   0   B. Needle thoracostomy
   0   C. Placing the patient on a pulse oximeter
   0   D. Obtaining a chest x-ray film

21. Based on the emergency nurse's initial assessment of this patient, the primary nursing diagnosis would be:

   0   A. Injury, potential for

   0   B. Fluid volume deficit

   0   C. Activity intolerance

   0   D. Gas exchange, impaired

22. After the emergency nurse performs the needle thoracostomy, evaluation of the effectiveness of this procedure would include all of the following *except:*

   0   A. A rush of air

   0   B. Improvement in the patient's blood pressure

   0   C. Increased shortness of breath

   0   D. Decreased shortness of breath

• • •

23. The classic signs and symptoms of a tension pneumothorax include all of the following *except:*

   0   A. Equal breath sounds bilaterally

   0   B. Tracheal deviation

   0   C. Distended neck veins

   0   D. Cyanosis

Cardiac contusion

A 19-year-old man was riding his bicycle and hit a hole in the road at a high rate of speed. He struck his chest on the ground. On arrival in the emergency department, the patient is alert and is complaining of chest pain. His vital signs are stable, but the rescue squad reports that the patient's pulse is irregular.

24. Because of the mechanism of injury, the initial assessment of this patient should include assessment for the presence of:

   0   A. Chest wall ecchymoses

   0   B. Head lacerations

   0   C. Orthopedic injuries

   0   D. Abdominal abrasions

25. An important intervention in the care of this patient would be:

   0   A. Monitoring and treating cardiac dysrhythmia

   0   B. Performing and documenting a Glasgow Coma Scale

0   C. Preparing the patient for hospitalization
0   D. Administering prescribed medications for pain

26. Because of the possibility of cardiac dysrhythmia in this patient, the nursing diagnosis the emergency nurse may base interventions on is:
0   A. Fluid volume deficit, potential
0   B. Infection, potential for
0   C. Skin integrity, impaired
0   D. Cardiac output, decreased

27. The patient continues to have frequent premature ventricular contractions (PVCs) and is given lidocaine, 50 mg, as an IV bolus. A continuous drip is maintained at the rate of 2 mg/min. The emergency nurse evaluates the patient for the presence of lidocaine toxicity by observing for:
0   A. The onset of seizures
0   B. The absence of ventricular dysrhythmia
0   C. Redness at the IV site
0   D. The presence of chest pains

Pulmonary contusion

An 18-year-old woman was an unrestrained backseat passenger in an automobile involved in a collision. The patient was thrown against the backseat. On arrival in the emergency department, she is awake and is complaining of chest pain. Her vital signs are blood pressure, 110/70; pulse, 90 and regular; and respiratory rate, 32.

28. All of the following signs and symptoms indicate a possible pulmonary contusion in this patient *except:*
0   A. A sucking chest wound
0   B. Dyspnea
0   C. Restlessness and agitation
0   D. The presence of severe chest injuries

29. Because of the mechanism of injury and bruising on the patient's chest, a pulmonary contusion is suspected. During the initial management of this patient, the emergency nurse should:
0   A. Give the patient a fluid bolus to keep her blood pressure above 120/80
0   B. Prepare the patient for elective intubation to maintain an oxygen saturation of 98%

    0   C. Limit fluids unless the patient develops hypovolemia from an associated injury

    0   D. Administer 3 L of oxygen by nasal cannula

30. Based on the medical diagnosis given to this patient, the emergency nurse would base care on which of the following nursing diagnoses?

    0   A. Thought processes, altered, related to the patient's being admitted to the emergency department

    0   B. Gas exchange, impaired, related to the injury of the lung parenchyma from the pulmonary contusion

    0   C. Thermoregulation, ineffective, related to the patient's being trapped in the car for 30 minutes

    0   D. Activity intolerance related to the patient's chest injury

ANSWERS

1. **B. Assessment.** Retractions of the sternocleidomastoid muscle usually indicate severe asthma. This occurs because of increased air trapping, which forces the patient to use accessory muscles to lift the rib cage in order to generate higher negative pleural pressures.[2]

2. **C. Assessment.** Obtaining a PEF from the patient having an asthma attack will provide the emergency nurse with important information about the patient's pulmonary status. A PEF of less than 80 L/min indicates severe obstruction; a PEF of 80 to 200 L/min indicates moderate obstruction. The PEF can also be used to assess the effectiveness of the prescribed medical treatment the patient receives while in the emergency department. The PEF should be at least 15% over baseline after treatment or reach a minimum of 200 L/min.[8]

3. **C. Intervention.** A beta-agonist, which will cause bronchodilation, is used as the initial treatment of the asthmatic patient.[3] Frequently used beta-agonists include metaproterenol sulfate and albuterol.

4. **D. Analysis.** The inability to breathe, no matter what the cause, will generate anxiety. The emergency nurse will need to include interventions that will help decrease the patient's anxiety, as well as provide medication and physical comfort. A useful intervention would be structuring the environment so that the patient is not left alone. This can be done by placing the patient in a visible area of the department.[9]

5. **C. Evaluation.** All of the above except the blood gas results would indicate that the asthmatic patient may need to be intubated. If the patient

were unable to verbalize or cough, this would be an indication of severe distress that may need to be treated with intubation.[3]

6. **C. Assessment.** Bacteria that have been found to cause pneumonia include legionella, mycoplasma, and *Streptococcus pneumoniae.* AIDS can contribute to the patient's being at risk for developing pneumonia, but does not cause it.[8]

7. **B. Intervention.** The patient with pneumonia is at risk of becoming dehydrated. Providing fluids for these patients is an important nursing intervention.[10]

8. **A. Assessment.** When obtaining a history from a patient who is experiencing chest pain, the emergency nurse obtains information about the possible causes of the chest pain. A part of this history is identification of risk factors; recent surgery, immobility, trauma, use of oral contraceptives, pregnancy, and obesity are risk factors for pulmonary embolus.[11]

9. **A. Intervention.** Since the patient has suffered an acute pulmonary embolus, the initial treatment would include the administration of a direct-acting anticoagulant. Heparin calcium is a direct-acting anticoagulant because it activates antithrombin III and factor X^a, which neutralize thrombin.[7]

10. **B. Analysis.** Tissue perfusion, altered (cardiopulmonary), would be an appropriate nursing diagnosis. This condition is a result of the pulmonary emboli. Included in the signs and symptoms of this nursing diagnosis is the patient's low blood pressure. The initial care of this patient by the emergency nurse will be based on interventions to improve tissue perfusion.[4]

11. **D. Evaluation.** Heparin can cause all of the above complications, including in rare instances the actual formation of more clots, which may cause chest pain, neurological deficits, and diminished pulses in extremities.[6]

12. **B. Assessment.** The history and physical presentation of this child is strongly suggestive of epiglottitis. Because of the possibility of obstruction, the child's throat should not be examined until the child is in a safe environment that includes personnel capable of emergency airway management. The potential dangers of evaluating the child's throat include precipitating laryngospasm and complete obstruction leading to respiratory arrest.[12]

13. **D. Intervention.** When the child is suffering acute respiratory distress from epiglottitis, the first intervention is to prepare the child for intubation. Administration of antibiotics would come after airway stabilization. Administration of racemic epinephrine is not recommended for the child with epiglottitis because of the potential of laryngospasm.[5]

14. **B. Intervention.** According to the Basic Life Support Guidelines for Infant FBAO Management (Conscious) of the American Heart Association, the emergency nurse should determine airway obstruction, place the infant face down and deliver four back blows, and then turn the infant over on the back and deliver four thrusts in the midsternal region. This is repeated until the object is expelled or the infant becomes unconscious.[12]

15. **C. Evaluation.** As noted in the previous answer, an indication that these maneuvers are not effective would be the child's becoming unconscious.

16. **B. Assessment.** The most common item that is aspirated by the child under age 3 years is the hot dog.[5]

17. **A. Intervention.** The management of the child with asthma is based on obtaining bronchodilation. It has been shown recently that this can be done well with the use of a beta-agonist such as albuterol, terbutaline, or metaproterenol.[7]

18. **C. Evaluation.** An early indication of hypoxia in the infant is irritability. It is important for the emergency nurse to teach parents the signs and symptoms of early hypoxia so that there may be early intervention in the management of pediatric respiratory emergencies.[7]

19. **A. Assessment.** Following the formula of airway, breathing, and circulation, the emergency nurse would assess the patient's ability to maintain his airway. This patient is alert and able to speak but is complaining of shortness of breath. In assessing ventilation (breathing), the emergency nurse would auscultate for the presence or absence of breath sounds. Since one of the major interventions in the management of chest trauma is assuring adequate ventilation, the absence of breath sounds and the complaint of shortness of breath indicate the need for interventions to return adequate airflow.[13]

20. **B. Intervention.** Until a chest tube can be inserted to improve the patient's ventilation, the emergency nurse should prepare and perform a needle thoracostomy. Two areas can be used for a needle thoracostomy: the second intercostal space in the midclavicular line or the fifth intercostal space in the midaxillary line. A large-bore needle is used (14 gauge), and the area should be prepared with antiseptic solution; the needle is inserted on the injured side.[14]

21. **D. Analysis.** Once again based on the ABCs, the initial nursing diagnosis on which to establish nursing interventions would be impaired gas exchange. The emergency nurse's interventions would initially be directed at providing interventions to correct the injuries that are impairing the patient's gas exchange.

22. **C. Evaluation.** The purpose of a needle thoracostomy is to improve the symptoms of tension pneumothorax, which include shortness of breath and hypotension. If there is no improvement or the patient's shortness of breath increases, another needle may need to be placed. The needle may not have completely entered the chest cavity, or it may have become kinked.

23. **A. Assessment.** The signs and symptoms of a tension pneumothorax include tracheal deviation, respiratory distress, unilateral absence of breath sounds, distended neck veins, and cyanosis.[15]

24. **A. Assessment.** Since the mechanism of injury involves the patient striking his chest and the patient is complaining of chest pain, the emergency nurse should assess the patient for the presence of chest wall injury. This would include the presence of abrasions or contusions on the chest wall.[10]

25. **A. Intervention.** Cardiac contusions leave the patient at risk for the development of life-threatening injuries related to cardiac damage. The most important initial intervention based on the presence of an irregular pulse would be the monitoring and treatment of cardiac dysrhythmia.

26. **D. Analysis.** The patient with myocardial contusion may suffer decreased cardiac output for several reasons. First, damage to the myocardium may result in pericardial tamponade, valvular disruption, and coronary artery occlusion. In addition, the patient may also suffer cardiac dysrhythmia, such as premature ventricular contractions and ventricular tachycardia, and conduction abnormalities.[16]

27. **A. Evaluation.** There are many indications of lidocaine toxicity, including hypotension, bradycardia, drowsiness, dizziness, and seizures.[6]

28. **A. Assessment.** The signs and symptoms of pulmonary contusion include a high index of suspicion based on the mechanism of injury, dyspnea, an ineffective cough, restlessness and agitation, and the presence of other severe chest injuries.[17]

29. **C. Intervention.** If the patient does not have hypotension from another related injury, such as an abdominal injury, fluids should be restricted for the patient with a pulmonary contusion. Because of the injury to the patient's lungs, the patient is at risk for developing complications from fluid overload, such as ARDS and hypoxia. Diuretics and steroids may be considered for the treatment of these patients.[15]

30. **B. Analysis.** Because of the injury to the patient's lungs and the possibility of a pulmonary contusion, the patient's care should be based on keeping her oxygenated. Defining characteristics of this nursing diagnosis include

confusion, somnolence, restlessness, irritability, inability to move secretions, hypoxia, and hypercapnia.[18]

REFERENCES

1. Thompson JM et al: *Mosby's manual of clinical nursing,* ed 2, St Louis, 1989, Mosby–Year Book.
2. Barkin RM: Pediatric respiratory emergencies, *Emerg Care Q* 5:71, 1989.
3. Wolfe RE, Honigman B: Acute asthma in the emergency department, *Emerg Care Q* 5:37, 1989.
4. Martinez R: Foreword, *Emerg Care Q* 4:vii, 1988.
5. Barkin RM: Pediatric respiratory emergencies, *Emerg Care Q* 5:71, 1989.
6. Chameides L, editor: *Textbook of pediatric advanced life support,* Dallas, 1989, American Heart Association.
7. Karb VB, Queener SF, Freeman JB: *Handbook of drugs for nursing practice,* St Louis, 1989, Mosby–Year Book.
8. Cole JA, Plantz SH: *Emergency medicine,* New York, 1990, McGraw-Hill.
9. McFarland GK, McFarlane EA: *Nursing diagnosis and intervention: planning for patient care,* St Louis, 1989, Mosby–Year Book.
10. Huddleston SS, Ferguson SG: *Critical care and emergency nursing,* Springhouse, Pa, 1990, Springhouse.
11. Rea R et al: *Emergency nursing core curriculum,* ed 3, Philadelphia, 1987, WB Saunders.
12. Selbst SM: Epiglottitis. In Barkin RM, editor: *The emergently ill child,* Rockville, Md, 1987, Aspen.
13. Kuhlmann TP: Pulmonary injuries, *Emerg Care Q* 4:29, 1989.
14. Rea R, editor: *Trauma nursing core course,* Chicago, 1987, Emergency Nurses Association.
15. *Advanced trauma life support course,* Chicago, 1989, American College of Surgeons.
16. French RS: Myocardial contusion, *Emerg Care Q* 4:41, 1988.
17. Sheehy SB: *Mosby's manual of emergency care,* ed 3, St Louis, 1990, Mosby–Year Book.
18. Carlson JH et al: *Nursing diagnosis: a case study approach,* Philadelphia, 1991, WB Saunders.

Chapter 16

Shock Emergencies

REVIEW OUTLINE

I. Physiology
   A. Normal vital signs based on the patient's age and disease state
   B. Normal urinary output
   C. Neuroendocrine response in specific shock states: hypovolemic, cardiogenic, and septic
   D. Acid-base balance
   E. Cellular response in shock
      1. Oxygen consumption
         a. Aerobic metabolism
         b. Anaerobic metabolism
      2. Release of toxins from cellular damage
   F. Normal and abnormal hemodynamic readings
   G. Physical and psychoenvironmental assessment
II. Types of shock
   A. Hypovolemic
   B. Distributive shock
      1. Septic shock
      2. Anaphylactic shock
      3. Spinal shock
   C. Pump failure: cardiogenic shock
III. Collaborative care of the patient with a shock emergency
   A. Basic and advanced life support
   B. Need to correct oxygen deficit
      1. Intubation, hyperventilation
      2. Evaluation of perfusion
   C. Fluid resuscitation
      1. Colloid vs. crystalloid
      2. Administration of blood

    3. Autotransfusion

    4. Administration of blood components

    5. Disseminated intravascular coagulation (DIC)

  D. Identification and treatment of other injuries or disease states

  E. Medications

    1. Oxygen

    2. Pressor agents

    3. Steroids

    4. Naloxone

    5. Antibiotics

  F. Military antishock trousers (MAST) or pneumatic antishock garment (PASG)

    1. Indications

    2. Contraindications

    3. Applications

    4. Controversies

IV. Related nursing diagnoses

  A. Airway clearance, ineffective

  B. Cardiac output, decreased

  C. Fluid volume deficit

  D. Gas exchange, impaired

  E. Grieving

  F. Infection, potential for

  G. Injury, potential for

  H. Posttrauma response

  I. Tissue perfusion, altered

INTRODUCTION

Gross stated in 1872 that "shock is the rude unhinging of the machinery of life."[1] Shock is seen as basically a cellular phenomenon in which the cells do not receive adequate circulation for the exchange of oxygen, nutrients, and toxins. When the individual components of the body cannot function, the "whole" body will not function.[1]

Shock results from multiple origins, including hypovolemic, hemorrhagic, neurogenic, vasogenic, and septic. Many texts are available that address the pathophysiology of each of these types of shock, and some of these are listed in the References at the end of this chapter.

Throughout the past few decades, the early detection of shock, as well as its treatment, has changed and improved. However, the most effective treatment of shock remains prevention. One method of prevention that is used by the emergency nurse is recognition of the patient at risk, which is accomplished by performing a physical assessment that initially evaluates the patient's airway, breathing or respiratory effort, and circulation. In addition, assessment data such as orthostatic vital signs (when the patient's disease state or injuries allow them), core temperature, cardiac monitor, ECG, capillary refill, urinary output, and skin color and turgor can provide further information about the patient.

The patient's history is an important component in the "recognition" of shock. Why is the patient in the emergency department? Has the patient been injured in a motor vehicle crash? Has the patient been vomiting for several days? Does the patient have a Foley catheter or gastric tube in place, which may leave the patient at risk for developing sepsis? Often, the history can point the emergency nurse toward the origin of the patient's shock state.

The collaborative management of the patient who is in a shock state is based on basic and advanced life support. The origin of the shock needs to be quickly identified and corrected. For example, if the volume loss is from a ruptured spleen, surgical intervention may be required. Other methods used in the treatment of shock include the use of vasopressors, steroids, or antibiotics; insertion of central monitoring lines, arterial monitoring catheters, or Swan-Ganz catheters; and correction of hyperthermia.[1,2]

REVIEW QUESTIONS
Hypovolemic Shock

An 18-month-old girl is brought to the emergency department by her parents. They state that she has been vomiting and passing loose stools for 24 hours. She is becoming difficult to arouse and is irritable. The child's vital signs are blood pressure, 80/40; pulse, 180; respiratory rate, 46; and temperature (rectal), 101° F. The baby's skin turgor is poor.

1. During the initial assessment of this child, the emergency nurse should:
   0 A. Obtain a history of childhood immunizations
   0 B. Palpate central and peripheral pulses
   0 C. Perform a Denver Developmental evaluation
   0 D. Take the child immediately from the parents

2. The physician has ordered a fluid bolus of normal saline to help correct the patient's hypovolemia. The parents state that the child weighs 24

pounds. Using the fluid resuscitation formula of 20 ml/kg, how much fluid should the child be given?

0   A. 1000 ml of normal saline

0   B. 480 ml of normal saline

0   C. 230 ml of normal saline

0   D. 340 ml of normal saline

3. The initial emergency nursing care of this patient should be based on the following nursing diagnosis:

0   A. Fatigue

0   B. Fluid volume deficit

0   C. Growth and development, altered

0   D. Hyperthermia

4. The child is given the fluid bolus as ordered. Of the following, which will occur first if the fluid resuscitation is effective?

0   A. A decrease in the baby's hematocrit

0   B. Improvement in the baby's mental status

0   C. A decrease in the baby's peripheral pulses

0   D. An increase in rate of the baby's central pulses

Hemorrhagic Shock

A 24-year-old woman was an unrestrained driver in an automobile involved in a head-on collision. At the scene of the accident, her blood pressure was 88/60, her pulse was 120, and her respiratory rate was 24. MAST pants were placed by the paramedics, and all compartments have been inflated.

5. In addition to the initial advanced life support assessment, the emergency nurse should:

0   A. Obtain orthostatic vital signs when the patient arrives

0   B. Cut off the MAST pants as soon as the patient arrives

0   C. Start dextrose 5% in water (D_5W) for fluid resuscitation in both arms

0   D. Inspect the patient for sources of blood loss

6. Two large-bore IV lines are established, and after infusion of 2 L of Ringer's lactate solution, the patient's blood pressure is 100/60. The emergency physician has ordered that the MAST pants be deflated. The emergency nurse will deflate:

0   A. The left leg first

0   B. The right leg last
0   C. Both legs at once
0   D. The abdominal compartment first

7. An absolute contraindication to the use of MAST pants or PASG for the patient in shock is:
0   A. A head injury
0   B. Pregnancy
0   C. An abdominal injury
0   D. Pulmonary edema

8. Blood gases were obtained from this patient on arrival in the emergency department. The results were pH, 7.30; Po_2, 60; Pco_2, 38; and HCO_3, 18. The patient has a mask in place that is delivering 80% oxygen. Based on these blood gas results, the emergency nurse should plan interventions using the following nursing diagnosis:
0   A. Posttrauma response
0   B. Gas exchange, impaired
0   C. Fluid volume deficit
0   D. Fatigue

Cardiogenic Shock

A 72-year-old man comes to the emergency department complaining of severe midsternal chest pain and shortness of breath. He has been coughing up pink, frothy sputum. His blood pressure is 80 by palpation, his pulse is 120, and his respiratory rate is 32. His monitor shows sinus tachycardia with frequent multifocal premature ventricular contractions (PVCs).

9. The patient who develops cardiogenic shock has infarcted how much of his left ventricle?
0   A. Less than 10%
0   B. More than 40%
0   C. Less than 5%
0   D. Less than 40%

10. The emergency physician has ordered a dopamine drip to be started. The drip is to run at the rate of 5 µg/kg/min. The solution of drug available contains 1000 µg/ml. The patient weighs 90 kg. At what rate should the IV pump be set?
0   A. 12 ml/hr

O   B. 8 ml/hr
O   C. 63 ml/hr
O   D. 27 ml/hr

11. For the patient in cardiac shock, the emergency nurse would base care
    on the following nursing diagnosis:
    O   A. Fluid volume excess
    O   B. Fatigue
    O   C. Cardiac output, decreased
    O   D. Infection, potential for

12. The expected outcome of the collaborative care initiated for this patient is:
    O   A. Correction of hypotension
    O   B. Improvement in cardiac function
    O   C. Diminished cough
    O   D. Improvement in skin color

Septic Shock

*An elderly woman has been sent to the emergency department by a nursing home staff.
They state that the patient has been hyperventilating, is cold to the touch, and has a
rapid pulse. She has recently been treated for pneumonia with oral antibiotics. The
patient's initial vital signs are blood pressure, 90/60; pulse, 100; respiratory rate, 36;
and temperature (rectal), 97° F.*

13. Blood gases are drawn. The results are pH, 7.48; Po_2, 78; Pco_2, 20; and
    HCO_3, 22. She was receiving 4 L of oxygen when these were drawn.
    These gases indicate:
    O   A. Respiratory alkalosis
    O   B. Metabolic acidosis
    O   C. Respiratory acidosis
    O   D. Metabolic acidosis

14. Before administration of IV antibiotics, the emergency nurse should:
    O   A. Draw at least two blood specimens for culture and sensitivity
    O   B. Check the patient's core body temperature
    O   C. Assess the patient's skin for any swelling or rashes
    O   D. Administer antipyretics

15. A Foley catheter is inserted in the patient before fluid resuscitation is
    initiated. What criterion could the emergency nurse use to evaluate the
    effectiveness of the fluid resuscitation of this patient?

0   A. Urinary output of 10 ml/hr
0   B. Urinary output of 5 ml/hr
0   C. Urinary output of 20 ml/hr
0   D. Urinary output of 30 ml/hr

ANSWERS

1. **B. Assessment.** Based on the history given by the baby's parents of vomiting and loose stools, in addition to physical assessment data of a pulse of 180, a respiratory rate of 46, and increasing lethargy, the emergency nurse should consider that the patient may be in shock, which may be a result of fluid loss from vomiting and diarrhea. However, since young children normally have faster heart and respiratory rates and a lower blood pressure, evaluation of both the central and peripheral pulses would provide the emergency nurse with additional information about the patient's shock state.[3]

2. **C. Intervention.** Twenty-four pounds equals 11 kg, which is multiplied by 20 ml, equaling 230 ml of normal saline.

3. **B. Analysis.** Because the child is suffering from hypovolemic shock, the emergency nurse should base care on the nursing diagnosis of fluid volume deficit. Defining characteristics of this nursing diagnosis include decreased venous filling, increased temperature, hypotension, and increased pulse rate.[4]

4. **B. Evaluation.** Since the child has already been displaying signs and symptoms of hypoperfusion, monitoring for changes in the child's neurological status will give the emergency nurse the most immediate method with which to evaluate the effectiveness of the fluid bolus.[3]

5. **D. Assessment.** During the initial evaluation, identifying the source of bleeding is as important as stabilizing the patient's airway and breathing, because the bleeding needs to be controlled in order to correct the effects of the pathophysiology of shock.[1,2]

6. **D. Intervention.** The abdominal compartment is the first portion of the MAST pants or PASG to be deflated. Once this section has been deflated, a blood pressure reading should be obtained. If the patient's blood pressure suddenly falls again, the trousers are reinflated until more fluid is given or the hemorrhage is controlled by other means, such as surgical intervention.[5]

7. **D. Assessment.** Absolute contraindications to the use of MAST pants or PASG are pulmonary edema and circulatory instability secondary to myocardial insufficiency. MAST pants should be used with caution in penetrating injuries associated with intrathoracic hemorrhage, a ruptured diaphragm, or severe central nervous system injury.[6]

8. **B. Analysis.** The blood gas results demonstrate that the patient is hypoxic.

A defining characteristic of this nursing diagnosis is hypoxia, which is demonstrated by the blood gas results. Collaborative care needs to be directed at correcting the oxygen deficit.[4]

9. **B. Assessment.** The patient who is in cardiogenic shock has lost over 40% of the left ventricle from a massive infarct, direct trauma to the myocardium, or several infarcts.[2]

10. **D. Intervention.** The formula that would be used to calculate this answer is[7]:

$$\frac{(\text{Prescribed dose in } \mu g/kg/min) \ (60 \ min/hr) \ (kg \ body \ weight)}{(\mu g/ml \ solution)}$$

will equal ml/hr.

$$\frac{(5 \ \mu g/kg/min) \ (60 \ min/hr) \ (90 \ kg)}{1000 \ \mu g/ml} = 27 \ ml/hr$$

11. **C. Analysis.** The defining characteristics of decreased cardiac output include dysrhythmia; hypotension; cold, clammy skin; edema; dyspnea; jugular vein distention; and decreased urinary output.[4]

12. **B. Evaluation.** The expected outcome of the initial collaborative care of the patient in cardiogenic shock is improved cardiac function. This may be accomplished through a combination of medication and decreasing of stress on the heart.[2,5]

13. **A. Assessment.** An initial indication of septic shock is respiratory alkalosis and hypotension. It is important for the emergency nurse to note that this is an early sign so that prompt identification of septic shock and appropriate interventions can keep the patient from developing further complications.[2]

14. **A. Intervention.** At least two blood specimens should be obtained from two separate sites before IV antibiotics are initiated.[6]

15. **D. Evaluation.** Urinary output for this patient should be 30 ml/hr or greater. A decrease in output of 20 ml/hr would be a warning sign.[4,6]

REFERENCES

1. Vary T, Linberg S: Pathophysiology of traumatic shock. In Cardona V et al, editors: *Trauma nursing: from resuscitation through rehabilitation*, Philadelphia, 1988, WB Saunders.

2. Zoellner-Hunter J: Shock. In Kitt S, Kaiser J, editors: *Emergency nursing: a physiologic and clinical perspective*, Philadelphia, 1990, WB Saunders.

3. Chameides L: *Textbook of pediatric advanced life support*, Dallas, 1988, American Heart Association.

4. McFarland GK, McFarlane EA: *Nursing diagnosis and intervention: planning for patient care*, St Louis, 1989, Mosby–Year Book.

5. Committee on Trauma: *Advanced trauma life support*, Chicago, 1988, American College of Surgeons.

6. Thompson JM et al: *Mosby's manual of clinical nursing*, ed 2, St Louis, 1989, Mosby–Year Book.

7. Burns C, Crawford M: A method for rapidly calculating intravenous drip rates, *Focus Crit Care* 15:46-48, 1988.

Chapter 17 _____

Substance Abuse Emergencies

REVIEW OUTLINE

I. Effects of drugs on specific systems
   A. Cardiovascular: cardiac output and venous return
   B. Respiratory: depression
   C. Neurological: altered mental status
   D. Renal function
   E. Hepatic function
   F. Gastrointestinal function
   G. Acid-base balance

II. Collaborative care of the patient with a substance abuse emergency
   A. ABCs (airway, breathing, circulation)
   B. Removal of the substance
   C. History related to the incident
      1. What was taken
      2. When it was taken
      3. How it was taken (intravenously, intramuscularly, orally, inhaled)
   D. Past medical history
      1. Known medical problems
      2. History of previous substance abuse
      3. Allergies
   E. Initial management
      1. Airway: possibility of aspiration
      2. Breathing: possibility of respiratory depression
      3. Circulation: blood pressure, pulse, cardiac monitor
      4. Neurological assessment
         a. Level of consciousness
         b. Pupillary response

       c. Motor response

       d. Sensory response

    5. Respiratory assessment

    6. Cardiovascular assessment

  F. Therapeutic interventions

    1. Oxygen

    2. Naloxone, IV push

    3. Dextrose 50%

    4. Thiamine

    5. Ipecac

    6. Charcoal

    7. Cathartic to enhance excretion

    8. Gastric lavage

    9. Arterial blood gases

    10. Drug screen

III. Related nursing diagnoses

  A. Airway clearance, ineffective

  B. Breathing pattern, ineffective

  C. Cardiac output, decreased

  D. Coping, ineffective individual

  E. Fear

  F. Gas exchange, impaired

  G. Injury, potential for

  H. Poisoning, potential for

  I. Violence, potential for: self-directed or directed at others

IV. Specific substance abuse emergencies

  A. Alcohol

  B. Narcotics

    1. Heroin

    2. Methadone

    3. Oxycodone

    4. Codeine

    5. Meperidine

  C. Amphetamines

  D. Cocaine

  E. Hallucinogens

  F. Barbiturates

  G. Methaqualone (Quaalude)

  H. Ethchlorvynol (Placidyl)

  I. Others

1. Typewriter correction fluid
2. Glue
3. Propane

INTRODUCTION

Unfortunately, substance abuse has become a major problem in the United States. Drugs such as alcohol and cocaine cause many physical and psychological problems that are cared for in the emergency department.

There are several substances that are abused, including depressants, stimulants, hallucinogens, and analgesics. Some of these substances are illegal, whereas others, such as alcohol, can be obtained over-the-counter.[1]

The patient who is treated in the emergency department because of substance abuse presents a difficult challenge. Because these drugs affect the central nervous system, basic vital functions such as airway, breathing, and circulation may be impaired. In addition, when substances are used in relation to injury, these drugs can mask severe injury. It is important to always rule out an organic cause for the patient's altered mental and physical status before blaming the patient's condition entirely on the use of some type of substance.

There are both psychosocial and physical signs and symptoms of substance abuse. Psychosocial signs and symptoms associated with substance abuse include euphoria, emotional lability, impaired judgment, psychomotor agitation, impaired attention, irritability, delusions, and hallucinations. Physical signs and symptoms include tachycardia, hypertension, lack of coordination, constricted or dilated pupils, tremors, seizures, cold, clammy skin, slurred speech, and death.[1]

Alcohol

Alcohol is one of the most abused substances in the United States. Over 10 million people suffer from alcoholism in the United States, and 70% of the adult U.S. population have at least one drink during the year. Alcohol and other abused substances have cost the United States millions of dollars in lost work. Alcohol-related injuries and diseases cost millions of dollars in health care resources each year.[1,2]

The person who abuses alcohol will suffer central nervous system depression, interference with the thermoregulatory mechanism, gastric irritation, and liver and pancreatic damage. In large doses alcohol may cause coma and death.[3]

Hallucinogens

During the 1960s and 1970s the use of substances causing hallucinations was very popular. During the 1980s their use decreased, but two hallucinogenic substances still in use may be encountered by the emergency department nurse: phencyclidine (PCP) and lysergic acid diethylamide (LSD). Both drugs cause intense and dangerous visual and auditory hallucinations. In addition, both drugs may induce psychosis and elicit behavior that is dangerous not only to the patient, but to the emergency department staff as well.[4,5]

Cocaine

The use of cocaine has become one of the most popular "recreational" forms of substance abuse. It has been estimated that in the United States 30 million individuals have tried it and 5 million people regularly use it.[6] The source of cocaine is the *Ethroxylon coca,* a plant native to Peru, Bolivia, and Columbia. However, it is now cultivated in many Central American countries.

Cocaine is abused in many ways. The drug can be ingested nasally, as well as injected intravenously. A dried form of the drug known as "crack" is smoked.

Cocaine toxicity may cause seizures, as well as cardiovascular and respiratory collapse. The intoxicated patient will generally be talkative, physically active, and sociable, and may be slightly tachycardiac.

REVIEW QUESTIONS
Patient Assessment

A 16-year-old girl is brought to the emergency department by her parents. They state that she has been acting "funny" for several hours. Initial examination reveals that she is alert and oriented to person and is very agitated. Her vital signs are normal. When her parents are questioned about drug abuse by their daughter, they deny that she uses drugs, and a drug screen is obtained. The patient is admitted to the psychiatric unit for observation.

In the morning she is found to be unresponsive; her right pupil is fixed and dilated. An emergency computed tomography (CT) scan is obtained, and a large intraventricular bleed is found on her left side. She is transferred to another facility and later during the day is pronounced dead.

1. Additional information in the initial assessment of this patient should include:
   - 0   A. A history about any recent illnesses or injury
   - 0   B. Any drugs the patient has taken in the past

0   C. What type of family support systems are present
0   D. How the patient usually behaves in school

2. An important emergency nursing intervention in the care of the patient with altered mental status (such as in this case) would include obtaining a(n):
   0   A. Complete blood cell count (CBC)
   0   B. Blood glucose level
   0   C. ECG
   0   D. Drug screen

3. For the patient who is agitated (as in this case) or showing abusive behavior in the emergency department, the most appropriate nursing diagnosis would be:
   0   A. Anxiety
   0   B. Fear
   0   C. Violence, potential for: self-directed or directed at others
   0   D. Self-esteem, situational low

•   •   •

4. The effectiveness of emergency nursing interventions for the substance abuse patient with an altered mental status may be seen through:
   0   A. Improvement in blood drug levels
   0   B. Improvement in the level of consciousness
   0   C. Decreasing pharmacological restraints
   0   D. Removal of physical restraints

Alcohol Abuse

A 37-year-old man is brought to the emergency department complaining of severe abdominal pain, vomiting, and tremors. He admits to a history of alcohol abuse and states that he has had nothing to drink for 72 hours.

5. The initial assessment of this patient should include assessment for signs and symptoms of:
   0   A. Esophageal varices
   0   B. Malabsorption syndrome
   0   C. Delirium tremens
   0   D. Hypothermia

6. The patient begins grand mal seizure activity. The drug of choice to manage alcoholic seizures is:

0   A. Lidocaine, IV push
0   B. Phenobarbital, IV push
0   C. Phenytoin, IV push
0   D. Diazepam, IV push

7. Emergency nursing care for the alcoholic patient having a seizure is based on which of the following nursing diagnoses?
0   A. Sensory/perceptual alterations
0   B. Self-esteem disturbance
0   C. Injury, potential for
0   D. Nutrition, altered: less than body requirements

Hallucinogens

A man in his thirties is dropped off at the emergency department by his friends, who state that he has taken some PCP. The patient is alert and is screaming and kicking.

8. What physical finding could confirm that the patient ingested PCP?
0   A. Dilated pupils
0   B. Nystagmus
0   C. Muscle fasciculations
0   D. Hyperventilation

9. Emergency nursing care of the patient who has ingested a hallucinogen would include:
0   A. Provision of a safe and quiet environment
0   B. Notification of the authorities
0   C. Administration of a specific antidote
0   D. Patient referral for psychiatric care

10. The nursing diagnosis on which the preceding intervention would be based is:
0   A. Self-esteem disturbance
0   B. Knowledge deficit
0   C. Poisoning, potential for
0   D. Sensory/perceptual alterations (visual, auditory)

Cocaine Abuse

A 32-year-old woman complaining of severe chest pain after having smoked crack is brought to the emergency department by the rescue squad. She is alert, oriented, and extremely agitated. Her blood pressure is 200/100, her pulse rate is 130, and her pupils are constricted.

11. The initial assessment of this patient should include a(n):
    0   A. ECG
    0   B. Arterial blood gas determination
    0   C. Drug screen
    0   D. Dextrostick

12. During the initial assessment the patient's monitor shows ventricular tachycardia. A pulse is palpated. What drug should the emergency nurse prepare to give?
    0   A. Bretylium, 10 mg/kg IV push
    0   B. Procainamide, 50 mg IV push
    0   C. Lidocaine, 1 mg/kg
    0   D. Phenytoin, 50 mg IV push

13. The nursing diagnosis on which the emergency nurse would base care for this patient is:
    0   A. Cardiac output, decreased
    0   B. Poisoning, potential for
    0   C. Sensory/perceptual alterations (visual, auditory)
    0   D. Injury, potential for

Narcotic Abuse

A 30-year-old man is dropped off at the front lobby of the emergency department. He is apneic and has a pulse of 60 beats per minute. The patient has multiple "tracks" on both arms.

14. A common neurological finding in the patient who has taken a narcotic overdose is:
    0   A. Fixed and dilated pupils
    0   B. Unequal pupils
    0   C. Pinpoint pupils
    0   D. Nonreactive pupils

15. The initial dose of naloxone administered by the emergency nurse would be:
    0   A. 0.4 mg IV push
    0   B. 2 mg IV push

0 C. 1 g IV push
0 D. 0.2 mg IV push

ANSWERS

1. **A. Assessment.** When the history is not clear as to why a person is behaving in a certain way, it is important to rule out an organic or physical cause for a behavior change. When the patient's parents are questioned, it is discovered that their child had been complaining about severe headaches a few days before her behavior changed.
2. **B. Intervention.** All of these laboratory values would offer useful information about the patient's altered mental status; however, changes in the blood glucose level, particularly in the case of hypoglycemia, are manifested by an altered mental status and can be easily treated.
3. **C. Analysis.** The most appropriate diagnosis for the agitated or abusive patient in the emergency department is violence, potential for: self-directed or directed at others. Using this nursing diagnosis, the emergency nurse would provide care that not only protected the patient, but the rest of the emergency department staff as well.
4. **B. Evaluation.** Since these substances affect the central nervous system, improvement in the level of consciousness would offer a useful evaluative criteria.
5. **C. Assessment.** The most acute alcoholic emergency the emergency department nurse will have to care for is delirium tremens, which usually occur 72 hours after the patient's last drink. The symptoms of delirium tremens include confusion, disorientation, hallucinations, diaphoresis, and elevated temperature.[1]
6. **D. Intervention.** Diazepam is the fastest-acting drug that is used in the initial treatment of alcoholic withdrawal seizures. Diazepam crosses the blood-brain barrier more quickly than either phenobarbital or phenytoin.[7]
7. **C. Analysis.** Seizure activity places the patient at tremendous risk for injury. The emergency nursing care is directed at protecting the patient from injury related to the consequences of seizures, such as aspiration, anoxia, and falling.
8. **B. Assessment.** Nystagmus has been found to be a common neurological sign of PCP toxicity.[5]
9. **A. Intervention.** The initial care of the patient who has ingested a hallucinogen is to provide a safe and quiet environment for the patient. The effects of PCP generally last 48 hours.[5] The effects of LSD are patient

dependent.[6] Until the drug has worn off, the patient is at risk not only for self-injury, but for injury to the staff as well.

10. **D. Analysis.** Providing a safe and quiet environment would be based on the nursing diagnosis of sensory/perceptual alterations (visual, auditory). The majority of hallucinations associated with these drugs are visual and auditory. A safe, quiet environment will help decrease stimuli that may trigger more hallucinations. For severe hallucinations, sedation may be necessary.

11. **A. Assessment.** Cocaine in high doses may cause myocardial infarction. Because the patient is already complaining of severe chest pain, an ECG should be obtained to evaluate any cardiac complications and possible infarction related to the crack use.

12. **C. Intervention.** The first drug to be used, based on advanced cardiac life support (ACLS) standards, would be lidocaine, 1 mg/kg.

13. **A. Analysis.** The initial care of this patient would be based on the nursing diagnosis of cardiac output, decreased. This patient's immediate problem is her cardiac dysrhythmia, which needs to be treated according to ACLS protocol.

14. **C. Assessment.** Pinpoint pupils are a common neurological finding in the patient who has taken a narcotic overdose. In addition, the patient may be apneic and hypotensive.[8]

15. **B. Intervention.** The initial dose of naloxone is 2 mg IV push, which is followed, if needed, by an infusion of 0.4 mg/hr.[8]

REFERENCES

1. Thompson JM et al: *Mosby's manual of clinical nursing,* ed 2, 1989, St Louis, Mosby–Year Book.
2. Rea RE et al: *Emergency nursing core curriculum,* ed 3, Philadelphia, 1987, WB Saunders.
3. Litovitz T: The alcohols: ethanol, methanol, isopropanol, ethylene glycol, *Pediatr Clin North Am* 33:311-323, 1986.
4. Haddad L, Winchester J: *Clinical management of poisoning and drug overdose,* Philadelphia, 1983, WB Saunders.
5. Merrigan KS, Roberts JR: *LSD,* clinical paper, University of Cincinnati, Department of Emergency Medicine, 1986.
6. Higgins R: Cocaine abuse: what every nurse should know, *JEN* 15:318-323, 1989.
7. Karb VB, Queener SF, Freeman JB: *Handbook of drugs for nursing practice,* St Louis, 1989, Mosby–Year Book.
8. Sheehy SB: *Mosby's manual of emergency care,* ed 3, St Louis, 1990, Mosby–Year Book.

Chapter 18

Surface Trauma Emergencies

REVIEW OUTLINE

I.   Anatomy of the integumentary system
    A. Largest organ system of the body
    B. Epidermis
       1. Avascular
       2. Composed primarily of epithelial cells
       3. Responsible for regeneration of skin
    C. Dermis
       1. Composed of connective tissue, fibroblasts, microphages, and fat cells
       2. Vascular
       3. Has lymph channels and nerves
    D. Hypodermis
       1. Contains subcutaneous tissues
       2. Contains smooth muscle, the areolar bed, blood vessels, and nerves

II. Function of the skin
    A. Protection
    B. Temperature control
    C. Excretion of salt and water
    D. Preservation of body fluids
    E. Production of vitamin D

III. Process of wound healing
    A. Injury
    B. Vasoconstriction
       1. Sludging of blood
       2. Redness and swelling
    C. Epithelial cell migration
    D. Collagen replacement

IV.   Assessment of the integumentary system
    A. History
        1. Mechanism of injury
        2. Time when injury occurred
        3. Possibility of contamination
        4. Amount and type of bleeding
        5. Presence or absence of pain
        6. Numbness or tingling distal to the injury
        7. Previous interventions prior to arrival in the emergency department
    B. Past medical history
        1. Diabetes
        2. Cardiovascular disease
        3. Dermatological problems
        4. Medications
            a. Aspirin
            b. Immunosuppressants
            c. Steroids
            d. Anticoagulants
    C. Tetanus status
    D. Psychosocial history
    E. Age of the patient
    F. Inspection
        1. Edema
        2. Redness
        3. Presence of foreign bodies
        4. Extent of damage to the skin
    G. Neurovascular assessment
        1. Flexion
        2. Extension
        3. Palpation of distal pulses
        4. Sensation
        5. Two-point discrimination
V.   Collaborative care of the patient with surface trauma
    A. ABCs (airway, breathing, circulation)
    B. Control of bleeding
    C. Goals of wound care
        1. Prevention of infection
        2. Promotion of rapid healing
        3. Prevention of scarring
    D. Wound care

     1. Assessment of the wound
     2. Assessment of the patient's neurovascular status
     3. Cleansing of the wound
     4. Irrigation of the wound
     5. Anesthesia
     6. Hair removal *(never shave eyebrows)*
     7. Closure
        a. Sutures
        b. Staples
        c. Steri-strip
     8. Suture, staple, Steri-strip removal
     9. Dressing application
    10. Discharge instructions
  E. Medications
     1. Tetanus
     2. Antibiotics
     3. Rabies prophylaxis
VI. Related nursing diagnoses
  A. Anxiety
  B. Infection, potential for
  C. Fluid volume deficit
  D. Knowledge deficit
  E. Pain
  F. Skin integrity, impaired
VII. Specific surface trauma emergencies
  A. Abrasion
  B. Abscess
  C. Avulsion
  D. Contusion
  E. Puncture wound
  F. Bites
     1. Human
     2. Dog
     3. Cat
     4. Skunk
     5. Bat
     6. Fox
     7. Snake
     8. Insect
     9. Spider
    10. Aquatic animal

INTRODUCTION

T
he skin, or integument, is the largest organ system of the body. Its functions are protection, control of body temperature, primary sensation, excretion of water and salt, preservation of body fluids, and production of vitamin D. Injuries to the skin, or integumentary system, are a common reason why patients come to the emergency department. There are many sources of these injuries, including thermal or chemical sources, punctures (or penetrating trauma), lacerations, and abrasions.[1] This chapter focuses on some of the most common types of surface trauma seen in the emergency department.

The emergency collaborative care of the patient who has suffered an injury to the integumentary system includes the prevention of infection, promotion of rapid healing, and prevention of scarring.[2] Proper cleansing of the wound is important in the prevention of infection.[3] There are many types of solutions that can be used to cleanse a wound, including povidone-iodine, chlorhexidine, and pluronic-F-68. In addition, irrigation of the wound with sterile water or normal saline helps to remove debris and contaminants.[3]

Whenever the skin has been penetrated, the tetanus status of the patient should be evaluated. There are several recommendations available for the administration of tetanus, including recommendations from both the American College of Surgeons and the American College of Emergency Physicians. Recommendations for tetanus prophylaxis are also given in tabular form in a text by Kitt and Kaiser.[4]

Specific interventions, such as suturing or stapling, are determined by the type of wound, the time when the wound occurred, and the extent of injury caused by the wound. Surface injuries older than 6 hours are generally considered contaminated and may not be closed the same as a wound that occurred earlier.

Bites and Stings

Bites and stings, a frequent cause of surface trauma, not only produce trauma to the integumentary system, but may also contribute to injuries of the musculoskeletal and neurovascular systems of the body. In addition, bites and stings may also contribute to both local and systemic reactions from toxins that are introduced to the body through the injury.

Mechanical trauma may result from the pressure inflicted during the biting process, producing lacerations and puncture wounds. Bites and stings can contribute to the injection of injurious substances. The injection of some of these substances in already sensitized individuals may cause serious problems and even death from anaphylaxis. Bites and stings allow the skin to be damaged; thus organisms can invade the body. Some of the organisms found in bite and puncture wounds include *Pasteurella multocida, Enterobacter, Pseudomonas, Staphylococcus aureus,* streptococci, tetanus, and rabies. (It is interesting to note that 42 species of organisms have been cultured from the human mouth.[5-7]) Finally, patients may suffer from reactions to retained parts when bitten or stung. For example, the stinger may remain from a bee or yellow jacket.

Complications from bites include both systemic and local reactions. Some of these complications are cellulitis, lymphangitis, abscess formation, tenosynovitis, and transmission of diseases such as syphilis, tuberculosis, hepatitis, Lyme disease, and rabies.

Depending on what or who is inflicting the injury, bites and stings can occur all over one's body. Human bites, which frequently occur in fights and during sexual assault, may be inflicted on the upper extremities: the face, ears, nose, lower lip, and cheeks.[3] Insect, spider, and snake bites are more likely to occur on the lower extremities, such as the feet, legs, and ankles. Spider bites may occur on hands if one reaches into common hiding places for spiders, such as woodpiles.[1]

• • •

The review questions presented in this chapter encompass several different examples of sources of surface trauma and the treatment of the complications that can occur.

REVIEW QUESTIONS
Human Bites

1. The most frequently used antibiotic to treat a potential infection resulting from a human bite is:
   0   A. Penicillin
   0   B. Tetracycline
   0   C. Cephalosporin
   0   D. Erythromycin

2. A 25-year-old man comes to the emergency department complaining of an injury to his right hand. The patient states that he sustained the injury while punching someone in the mouth. On evaluation, a large laceration is found over the volar surface of his hand near the fifth digit. Initial care of this wound would include all of the following *except:*
   0   A. Copious irrigation of the wound
   0   B. Primary closure of the laceration

0   C. Administration of IV antibiotics
0   D. Administration of a tetanus shot

Insect Bites

3. A critical reaction to an insect bite or sting is:
   0   A. Anaphylaxis
   0   B. Cellulitis
   0   C. Serum sickness
   0   D. Erythema

4. The drug that is initially used in the treatment of anaphylaxis is:
   0   A. Diphenhydramine, 50 mg IV push
   0   B. Methylprednisolone, 125 mg IV push
   0   C. Epinephrine 1:1000, 0.3 mg subcutaneously
   0   D. Epinephrine 1:10,000, 0.3 mg subcutaneously

5. In addition to treating the patient with medications, what other nursing care is given to the patient in anaphylactic shock?
   0   A. Removal of the antigen
   0   B. Washing the wound with soap and water
   0   C. Giving the patient a tetanus shot
   0   D. Placing ice on the affected area

Spider Bites

6. The venom of the black widow spider is:
   0   A. Hemolytic
   0   B. Neurotoxic
   0   C. Nonpoisonous
   0   D. The cause of localized reactions

7. The most common drug used in the treatment of black widow spider bite envenomation is:
   0   A. Calcium chloride
   0   B. Epinephrine
   0   C. Calcium gluconate
   0   D. Sodium bicarbonate

8. The distinctive marking(s) of the brown recluse spider is (are):
   0   A. An "hour glass" on its abdomen
   0   B. Two-inch fangs

0   C. Its black and orange coloring
0   D. A "fiddle" on its back

9. The venom of the brown recluse spider can cause all of the following
   except:
   0   A. Tissue infarction and necrosis
   0   B. Fever
   0   C. Scarlatiniform rash
   0   D. Paralysis

Lyme Disease

Lyme disease is a relatively new disease that is transmitted by a tick bite. It was first identified in the middle 1970s and now has been reported in 44 states and on three continents.[5,8]

10. A sign or symptom of the first stage of Lyme disease is:
    0   A. Meningitis
    0   B. Cardiac dysrhythmia
    0   C. A ringlike rash
    0   D. Arthritis

11. The treatment of choice in the *early* stages of Lyme disease is:
    0   A. Penicillin, 20 to 24 million units daily IV
    0   B. Doxycycline, 100 mg b.i.d. PO
    0   C. Erythromycin, 250 mg q.i.d. PO
    0   D. Methylprednisolone, 125 mg IV

Snake Bites

12. A pit viper can be identified by all of the following *except:*
    0   A. Round pupils
    0   B. Elliptical pupils
    0   C. Thermoreceptor pits
    0   D. Triangular-shaped head

13. The initial management of a victim who has been bitten by a snake
    should include:
    0   A. Making an incision around the wound
    0   B. Immobilizing the affected part
    0   C. Applying a tourniquet
    0   D. Packing the affected area in ice

14. Sensitivity to which of the following can put a patient at greater risk of anaphylaxis during antivenin administration?

   0 A. Penicillin

   0 B. Epinephrine

   0 C. Horse serum

   0 D. Diphenhydramine

Mammalian Bites

15. Of the following, which animal is most likely to transmit rabies?

   0 A. Dog

   0 B. Cat

   0 C. Squirrel

   0 D. Skunk

16. A 15-year-old boy is brought to the emergency department by his parents after having been bitten by a bat. After cleansing and irrigating the wound, the emergency physician orders rabies prophylaxis to be initiated. The physician orders rabies immunoglobulin (RIG) (given in a dose of 20 IU/kg) and human diploid cell vaccine (HDCV). The patient's weight is 135 pounds. What is the dose of RIG to be given?

   0 A. 500 IU

   0 B. 1200 IU

   0 C. 600 IU

   0 D. 2400 IU

17. RIG is administered by:

   0 A. Giving an IV push after administering diphenhydramine and methylprednisolone

   0 B. Injecting one half the dose around the wound and giving the other half deep IM

   0 C. Injecting the total dose deep IM

   0 D. Giving half the dose IV and the other half deep IM

Abrasions and Lacerations

18. An 18-year-old man comes to the emergency department complaining of abrasions to both his thighs. The patient states that he was riding his motorcycle and lost control, scraping his legs on the road. Physical examination reveals that the patient has large abrasions on the tops of both of his thighs. A wound complication common to abrasions is:

   0 A. A large loss of fluids from the skin

0   B. Contamination of the wound by debris
0   C. Open wounds to the bone
0   D. Loss of sensation to the injured area

19. Contamination of an abrasion by asphalt may leave a patient at risk for:
0   A. The development of a third-degree burn from the asphalt
0   B. An anaphylactic reaction to the asphalt
0   C. Tattooing from retained asphalt
0   D. Development of tetanus from the asphalt

20. A 20-year-old woman comes to the triage nurse complaining of a severe laceration on her right wrist. The patient states that she tripped and put her hand through a plate glass door. The patient has a towel wrapped around the extremity. She is pale and diaphoretic. Her blood pressure is 90/60, and her pulse is 120. The initial care of this patient should be based on which of the following nursing diagnoses?
0   A. Fluid volume deficit related to blood loss from the wrist laceration
0   B. Skin integrity, impaired, related to the wrist laceration
0   C. Pain related to the wrist laceration
0   D. Anxiety related to the potential for disfigurement from the wrist laceration

ANSWERS

1. **C. Intervention.** Penicillin was used for a long time to treat the potential infection that may occur with human bites. However, cephalosporin has been found to be more effective. The initial dose should be given intravenously. In addition, if the patient is discharged, follow-up within 24 to 48 hours after injury is mandatory.[2]

2. **B. Intervention.** Primary closure of human bites is not recommended because of the potential for serious infection. The exception to this may be the face and the neck. The wound should be copiously irrigated, and any devitalized tissue should be debrided.[2]

3. **A. Assessment.** The reaction that will cause the most serious complications, and possibly death, is anaphylaxis. Anaphylactic shock is the result of an antigen-antibody reaction. Bee stings can frequently cause this response in a sensitized person.[9]

4. **C. Intervention.** The initial drug given to the patient in anaphylactic shock is epinephrine 1:1000, 0.3 mg subcutaneously.[6]

5. **A. Intervention.** The source of the toxin causing the systemic reaction

needs to be removed, and absorption of further antigen needs to be prevented.[10]

6. **B. Assessment.** The venom of the black widow spider is neurotoxic and is considered to be one of the most potent venoms secreted by an animal. Signs and symptoms of toxicity include muscle fasciculation, abdominal cramping, paralysis, and respiratory arrest.[5]

7. **C. Intervention.** Calcium gluconate provides muscle relaxation in doses of 10 ml of 10% solution. Other drugs that may be used in the treatment of black widow spider envenomation include antivenin, diazepam, and methocarbamol.[5]

8. **D. Assessment.** The brown recluse spider is also known as the "violin" or "fiddleback" spider. These spiders are large — up to 5 cm in length — and are usually dark brown to yellow in color.[1]

9. **D. Assessment.** Brown recluse venom produces both local and systemic reactions. Local reactions include the formation of necrotic lesions at the bite area. Systemic reactions include chills, fever, rash, disseminated intravascular coagulation (DIC), and death.[5]

10. **C. Assessment.** During the first stage of Lyme disease, a ringlike rash (called erythema chronicum migrans) will appear. This occurs 2 days to 2 weeks after inoculation by the spirochete.[5,7,8]

11. **B. Intervention.** Currently, early treatment of Lyme disease is doxycycline, 100 mg twice a day.[5,8]

12. **A. Assessment.** Identifying features of a pit viper include its elliptical pupils, a thermoreceptor pit located between its eyes and nostrils, and a triangular-shaped head.[5]

13. **B. Intervention.** In addition to stabilizing the patient's ABCs, immobilization of the bitten extremity has been found to be one of the best methods of preventing further absorption of the venom.[5]

14. **C. Assessment.** Antivenin is prepared from the serum of hyperimmunized horses. Sensitivity to horse serum, a history of hay fever, and urticaria can place a patient at greater risk for developing complications during administration of antivenin.[5]

15. **D. Assessment.** Animals at high risk for transmitting rabies include bats, skunks, foxes, bobcats, raccoons, and coyotes.[5]

16. **B. Intervention.** The dosage is 20 IU/kg; the patient's weight is 60 kg.[1]

17. **B. Intervention.** The recommended administration of RIG is to inject one half the dose around the wound and give the remaining half deep IM.[5]

18. **B. Assessment.** Abrasions result from the skin being forced against a hard surface, such as a road. Injury can occur to both the epidermis and

the dermis. The resultant injury is similar to a burn. Often, because of the mechanism of injury, these wounds are contaminated.[2,3]

19. **C. Assessment.** Asphalt is one of the most common contaminants found in an abrasion. If the abrasion is not properly cleansed and debrided, tattooing can occur because of the dark color of the asphalt. This can be especially disfiguring when the abrasion is on the patient's face.[2,3]

20. **A. Analysis.** Based on the initial assessment of this patient, the triage nurse's care would be based on the nursing diagnosis of fluid volume deficit related to blood loss from the wrist laceration.

REFERENCES

1. Genge M: Surface trauma. In Kitt S, Kaiser J, editors: *Emergency nursing: a physiologic and clinical perspective,* Philadelphia, 1990, WB Saunders.
2. Trott AT: *Wounds and lacerations: emergency care and closure,* ed 2, St Louis, 1991, Mosby–Year Book.
3. Trott AT: *Principles and techniques of minor wound care,* New York, 1985, Medical Examination Publishing.
4. Kitt S, Kaiser J, editors: *Emergency nursing: a physiologic and clinical perspective,* Philadelphia, 1990, WB Saunders.
5. Stewart C: *Environmental emergencies,* Baltimore, 1990, Williams & Wilkins.
6. Legge M, Murphy M: Human bite wounds, *JEN* 16:146-150, 1990.
7. Parker F: The skin and the elements: sun, plants, and stinging and biting organisms, *Emerg Care* 4:21-31, 1988.
8. Paparone P: The summer scourge of Lyme disease, *Am J Nurs* 6:44-47, 1990.
9. Sheehy S: *Mosby's manual of emergency care,* ed 3, St Louis, 1990, Mosby–Year Book.
10. Zull D: Anaphylaxis. In Kitt S, Kaiser J, editors: *Emergency nursing: a physiologic and clinical perspective,* Philadelphia, 1990, WB Saunders.

Chapter 19 _____

Toxicological Emergencies

REVIEW OUTLINE

I. General management of the patient with a toxicological emergency
    A. ABCs (airway, breathing, circulation)
        1. Assure a patent airway
        2. Monitor for respiratory changes
        3. Place the patient on a cardiac monitor
        4. Establish a large-bore intravenous line
        5. Insert a Foley catheter when indicated
    B. Termination of the toxicological exposure
        1. Remove the victim from the toxic environment
        2. Determine how the patient was exposed to the toxin (orally, intravenously, through the skin)
        3. Decontaminate the patient when indicated
        4. Induce vomiting when indicated (current research continues to demonstrate that this may become an obsolete practice)
        5. Perform gastric lavage when ordered
        6. Record the amount of emesis and a description of the emesis, saving a sample
        7. Administer a specific antidote when indicated
        8. Administer naloxone, dextrose 50% (D_{50}), thiamine, and oxygen
        9. Administer charcoal to neutralize the poison
        10. Administer a cathartic to enhance excretion of the toxin
II. History related to the toxicological emergency
    A. What was the patient exposed to or what did the patient take
    B. When was it taken
    C. What route (intravenous, intramuscular, oral, inhaled)
        1. Presence of tracts
        2. Scars
        3. Skin pops

    D. What interventions have been done before admission to the emergency
department

    E. Has the patient done this before

    F. Patient's past medical history

    G. Allergies

    H. Medications

    I. History of psychological problems

    J. History of abuse

III. Identification of the toxin

    A. Presence of burns around or in the mouth

    B. Odor of the patient's breath

    C. Eyes

        1. Pinpoint pupils: narcotics, chloral hydrate, phenothiazine, insecticides

        2. Dilated pupils: alcohol, amphetamines, cocaine, tricyclics

        3. Nystagmus: vertical, horizontal

    D. Vital signs

        1. Bradycardia: beta-blockers, digitalis toxicity, organophosphate poisoning

        2. Tachycardia: tricyclics, cocaine and crack, amphetamines, hallucinogens

    E. Neurological assessment

        1. Mental depression

        2. Excitability

        3. Pupillary changes

        4. Extraocular eye movements

        5. Changes in respiratory patterns

IV. Collaborative care of the patient with a toxicological emergency

    A. ABCs

        1. Assure a patent airway

        2. Arterial blood gases

        3. Cardiac monitor

        4. Large-bore intravenous line

        5. Specific antidote when available

        6. Neurological assessment

        7. Terminate toxic exposure

        8. Identify nature of the toxin

            a. Poisindex

            b. Poison Control Center

            c. Environmental Protection Agency (EPA)

            d. Local experts

      9. Gastric lavage

     10. Decontamination when indicated

     11. Foley catheter for accurate measurement of intake and output

     12. Administration of dextrose 50% (D_{50}), naloxone, thiamine, oxygen

     13. Administration of charcoal

     14. Administration of a cathartic

     15. Family assessment and care

V. Related nursing diagnoses

  A. Airway clearance, ineffective, related to toxic exposure

  B. Aspiration, potential for

  C. Breathing pattern, ineffective, related to toxic exposure

  D. Cardiac output, decreased, related to toxic exposure

  E. Coping, ineffective, related to a drug overdose

  F. Fluid volume deficit related to toxic exposure

  G. Gas exchange, impaired, related to toxic exposure

  H. Hyperthermia related to toxic exposure

  I. Injury, potential for, related to toxic exposure

  J. Knowledge deficit

  K. Poisoning, potential for

  L. Sensory/perceptual alterations related to toxic exposure

  M. Skin integrity, impaired, potential, related to toxic exposure

  N. Violence, potential for: self-directed or directed at others, related to toxic exposure

VI. Specific toxicological emergencies

  A. Drug overdoses and poisonings

     1. Acetaminophen

       a. Toxic amount

       b. Stages of toxicity

       c. Overdose management: *N*-acetylcysteine

     2. Salicylates

       a. Toxic amount

       b. Overdose management

     3. Amphetamines

     4. Alcohol

       a. Ethanol

       b. Methanol

     5. Barbiturates

     6. Benzodiazepines

     7. Caustic ingestions

     8. Cyanide

     9. Ethylene glycol

INTRODUCTION

*I*n 1989 there were 1,581,540 human poison exposures documented by the American Association of Poison Control Centers (AAPCC).[1] Furthermore, the majority of patients exposed to poison are evaluated and treated in the emergency department.

The review questions presented in this chapter offer examples of some of the most frequent types of poisonings seen by the emergency department nurse. The assessment, analysis, intervention, and evaluation components in the care of the poisoned patient are addressed.

Management of the Poisoned Patient

Supportive care is the key to management of the poisoned patient. Airway, ventilation, and circulatory maintenance are the mainstays of care of the poisoned patient. Unfortunately, compared with the number of poisons contained in the human environment, there are few antidotes known.

In addition to meeting the physical and physiological needs of the poisoned patient, the emergency nurse needs to provide emotional care. Particular attention needs to be given to why or how the patient was poisoned. Was it an environmental problem, an unintentional poisoning, or an intentional poisoning? It is important to assess whether the poisoning may have been a form of abuse, particularly if a child or elderly adult is involved.

Acetaminophen Poisoning

Acetaminophen is contained in many over-the-counter drugs. Its most popular name is Tylenol. Poisoning by acetaminophen can be very lethal. The drug, if not properly eliminated, can cause hepatic, renal, and cardiac failure. Ingestions of 7.5 g or 150 mg/kg are considered potentially toxic.

Salicylate Poisoning

Aspirin is the most common type of salicylate. It is one of the oldest nonprescription drugs used by humankind. As with acetaminophen, many over-the-counter drugs contain salycylates. There are three types of salicylate toxicity. Mild toxicity occurs with ingestions of less than 150 mg/kg, moderate toxicity occurs with ingestions of 150 to 300 mg/kg, and severe toxicity occurs with ingestions of 300 to 500 mg/kg.

Cyclic Antidepressant Poisoning

Antidepressants are used to treat depression in adults, nocturnal enuresis, and painful neuropathies in diabetic patients. In addition to tricyclic antidepressants, there are bicyclic and tetracyclic antidepressants. However, the most frequently prescribed antidepressants are tricyclic.[2]

The exact toxic level of poisoning cannot always be determined, because the drug accumulates in body tissues. The patient is treated according to the presenting symptoms. Cyclic antidepressants in toxic amounts induce the release of norepinephrine and then inhibit its reuptake, directly block alpha action, exert a quinidine-like effect on myocardial tissue, and cause atropine-like anticholinergic effects.[3] The most common cause of death in cyclic poisoning is related to cardiac toxicity. Signs and symptoms of cardiac toxicity include depression of myocardial contractility, prolongation of the QT interval, heart block, atrial and ventricular dysrhythmia, and sudden cardiac death.[3]

Hydrocarbon Poisoning

Hydrocarbons are contained in many substances that may be ingested, inhaled, or spilled directly onto the skin. Examples of hydrocarbons include gasoline, kerosene, turpentine, and camphor. The most common types of hydrocarbon poisoning seen by the emergency department nurse include ingestion of gasoline and kerosine and dermal exposure by these same substances.[4]

Hydrocarbon poisoning may cause pulmonary and cutaneous injuries. The major effects of ingestion of hydrocarbons are on the lungs, gastrointestinal tract, and central nervous system.[5]

Organophosphate Poisoning

Organophosphates are contained in many commercial insecticides. Their mechanism of action is achieved by their ability to combine with acetylcholinesterase. This causes increased salivation, vomiting, bronchospasm, bradycardia, muscle fasiculations, paralysis, ataxia, confusion, seizures, and coma.[6,7]

REVIEW QUESTIONS
Drug Overdose

A 20-year-old woman is brought to the emergency department by the rescue squad. Her mother states that the patient has been depressed and has been taking lorazepam (2 mg), which was prescribed by the family physician. An empty bottle, along with a bottle of wine, was found by her bed. Currently the patient is responding only to deep, painful stimuli.

1. The initial assessment of this patient would include which of the following?
   - 0   A. Consulting the toxicology file to find the antidote to lorazepam poisoning
   - 0   B. Determining the patient's ability to protect her airway
   - 0   C. Checking the patient's rhythm on the cardiac monitor
   - 0   D. Determining if the patient is suicidal

2. What would be the most appropriate intervention in the initial management of this patient?
   - 0   A. Insertion of an oral or nasopharyngeal airway tube
   - 0   B. Starting an IV infusion of dextrose 5% in water (D_5W) and administering D_{50} and naloxone
   - 0   C. Placing the patient on a cardiac monitor
   - 0   D. Administering ipecac

3. What would be an appropriate nursing diagnosis for this patient?
    - 0 A. Coping, ineffective individual, related to use of an antianxiety drug
    - 0 B. Poisoning, potential for, related to ingestion of an unknown amount of lorazepam and alcohol
    - 0 C. Family processes, altered, related to attempted suicide
    - 0 D. Infection, potential for, related to poisoning

4. The purpose of charcoal in the care of the poisoned patient is to
    - 0 A. Absorb toxins
    - 0 B. Induce vomiting
    - 0 C. Prevent cardiac dysrhythmia
    - 0 D. Decrease the possibility of bleeding after toxin ingestion

5. When obtaining a history of the patient who has taken an overdose (as in this case) or otherwise been poisoned, what additional information must the emergency department nurse obtain?
    - 0 A. The patient's medical history
    - 0 B. Any history of previous suicide attempts
    - 0 C. Any history of allergies
    - 0 D. Any present medications

Acetaminophen Poisoning

6. What is an important assessment parameter in the care of the patient who has ingested a toxic amount of acetaminophen?
    - 0 A. The serum acetaminophen level immediately following ingestion
    - 0 B. The serum acetaminophen level 24 hours after ingestion
    - 0 C. The serum acetaminophen level 4 hours after ingestion
    - 0 D. The serum acetaminophen level 48 hours after ingestion

7. What is the specific management of the patient who has a toxic acetaminophen level 4 or more hours after ingestion?
    - 0 A. Charcoal, 50 g
    - 0 B. Sodium bicarbonate, 1 mEq/kg
    - 0 C. Ipecac, 15 ml
    - 0 D. *N*-Acetylcysteine, 140 mg/kg

8. Which of the following assessment parameters may be used by the emergency department nurse to evaluate the toxicity of an acetaminophen poisoning?

0   A. Hepatic studies
0   B. Arterial blood gases
0   C. Coagulation studies
0   D. Electrolytes

Salicylate Poisoning

9. During the initial stages of salicylate poisoning, the blood gases may show:
0   A. Metabolic acidosis
0   B. Respiratory alkalosis
0   C. Respiratory acidosis
0   D. Metabolic alkalosis

10. In addition to gastric emptying and charcoal administration for the patient who has suffered salicylate poisoning, which of the following interventions may be useful?
0   A. Cardiac monitoring
0   B. Measuring intake and output
0   C. Alkaline diuresis
0   D. Inserting an arterial line

11. What nursing diagnosis would pertain to the patient who has been poisoned with salicylates?
0   A. Swallowing, impaired
0   B. Fluid volume deficit, potential
0   C. Family processes, altered
0   D. Infection, potential for

12. Because of the bleeding complications that may occur with salicylate poisoning, what laboratory value should the emergency department nurse evaluate?
0   A. Type and screen
0   B. BUN and creatinine level
0   C. Prothrombin time and partial thromboplastin time
0   D. Arterial blood gases

Cyclic Antidepressant Poisoning

13. A 3-year-old boy has ingested an unknown amount of his mother's amitriptyline. He is brought to the emergency department capable of protecting his airway and responding only to deep, painful stimuli. During the initial assessment of this patient, what would be a helpful assessment parameter to determine the amount of cyclic toxicity?

0   A. Level of consciousness
0   B. Capillary refill
0   C. Urinary output
0   D. Cardiac rhythm

14. The best method of preventing reabsorption in the management of cyclic poisoning is:

0   A. Gastric lavage
0   B. Administration of ipecac
0   C. Administration of sorbitol
0   D. Administration of charcoal

• • •

15. A pertinent nursing diagnosis for the patient who has been poisoned by cyclic antidepressants would be:

0   A. Noncompliance related to excessive ingestion of prescribed medications
0   B. Social isolation related to depression
0   C. Cardiac output, decreased, related to the quinidine-like effects of cyclic antidepressant toxicity
0   D. Injury, potential for, related to the effects of cyclic antidepressant poisoning

16. Because of the ability of cyclic antidepressants to block the reuptake of norepinephrine, what assessment parameter should be constantly evaluated by the emergency department nurse?

0   A. Temperature
0   B. Capillary refill
0   C. Blood pressure
0   D. Urinary output

Hydrocarbon Poisoning

A 1-year-old child has ingested an unknown amount of gasoline from an open container. He is awake, alert, and crying appropriately. He smells like gasoline. His respiratory rate is 30.

17. Because the patient has ingested a hydrocarbon, the initial assessment of this patient will be focused on his:

    0   A. Cardiac rhythm
    0   B. Respiratory system
    0   C. Gastrointestinal system
    0   D. Central nervous system

18. Because the child may be experiencing some respiratory distress, an appropriate emergency nursing intervention would be:
    0   A. Placing a temperature probe in the child
    0   B. Giving the child supplemental oxygen
    0   C. Placing the child in an isolation room
    0   D. Placing the child in a protective crib

19. A relevant nursing diagnosis in the care of this child would be:
    0   A. Injury, potential for, related to poisoning
    0   B. Gas exchange, impaired, related to pulmonary injury
    0   C. Cardiac output, decreased, related to hydrocarbon ingestion
    0   D. Aspiration, potential for, related to hydrocarbon ingestion

20. After 6 hours of observation in the emergency department, the child does not exhibit any signs or symptoms of injury from the gasoline ingestion. What additional information should be obtained by the emergency department nurse to evaluate the child's home environment?
    0   A. The number of siblings in the house
    0   B. The location of the gasoline and other possible toxins
    0   C. Who is responsible for the child's care
    0   D. The distance from the child's home to the emergency department

Organophosphate Poisoning

An elderly man attempted to commit suicide by locking himself in a closet and spraying himself with insecticide. On arrival in the emergency department, the patient is comatose and his monitor shows sinus bradycardia.

21. In addition to the initial assessment of the patient's airway, breathing, and circulatory status, the emergency nurse should also consider:
    0   A. The method of exposure to the poison
    0   B. The age of the patient
    0   C. Whether the patient is depressed
    0   D. Whether the patient may become violent

22. The drug of choice to reverse the toxic effects of organophosphate poisoning is:

0   A. Lidocaine, 1 mg/kg
0   B. Sodium bicarbonate, 1 mEq/kg
0   C. Atropine, 1 to 5 mg
0   D. Calcium chloride, 10 mg

23. An appropriate nursing diagnosis for this patient would be:
    0   A. Knowledge deficit related to the inappropriate use of an insecticide
    0   B. Coping, ineffective individual, related to depression
    0   C. Thought processes, altered, related to organophosphate poisoning
    0   D. Family processes, altered, related to age

24. What outcome in this patient would indicate the effectiveness of atropine in the treatment of organophosphate poisoning?
    0   A. Decreased salivation
    0   B. Increased bradycardia
    0   C. Increased ataxia
    0   D. Cardiopulmonary arrest

ANSWERS

1. **B. Assessment.** The most important component of the initial assessment of the poisoned patient is the patient's ability to protect his or her airway. Many poisons alter the patient's mental status, and the patient could quickly become at risk for aspiration, hypoventilation, and apnea.[8]

2. **A. Intervention.** The initial management of the poisoned patient is based on supportive management of airway, breathing, and circulation. Ipecac should not be given to a patient who is not capable of protecting his or her airway.[8]

3. **B. Analysis.** The most appropriate nursing diagnosis and one on which the emergency nurse could develop this patient's plan of care would be poisoning, potential for, related to ingestion of an unknown amount of lorazepam and alcohol. Because of the possible life-threatening complications that may occur with poisoning and the nature of the episodic care provided by the emergency department nurse, this particular diagnosis would encompass many of the relevant nursing actions that would be required by this patient.[9]

4. **A. Intervention.** Charcoal is a finely divided black powder with an extensive internal network of pores that absorb substances. For charcoal to be effective, it needs to be given as quickly as possible after ingestion of the toxic substance.[10] Recent research has suggested that in certain poisonings charcoal alone, rather than combined with the use of ipecac, may be useful in the initial treatment of the alert poisoned patient. It has been

found that many patients are unable to keep charcoal down until several hours after ipecac has been administered, thus being deprived of the charcoal's ability to absorb the poison.[3,11]

5. **B. Assessment.** In 1988 the AAPCC reported that 10% of human poisonings were intentional.[1] It is important to identify whether the patient has attempted suicide in the past to determine whether this particular incident was intentional or unintentional and to determine appropriate care for the patient, which might include a psychiatric evaluation.

6. **C. Assessment.** All patients should have a serum acetaminophen level drawn 4 hours after ingestion. The serum level immediately following ingestion will offer little information about the potential toxic level the patient may have ingested.[6]

7. **D. Intervention.** *N*-Acetylcysteine is indicated when the serum acetaminophen level remains at a toxic level after 4 hours or if an acetaminophen level cannot be obtained before 10 hours after ingestion. *N*-Acetylcysteine is given orally. It may cause vomiting and may have to be given through a nasogastric tube. It is interesting to note that research is currently being done on administering *N*-acetylcysteine intravenously.[6]

8. **A. Assessment.** Since acetaminophen poisoning is particularly toxic to the liver, baseline hepatic studies should be drawn. The peak hepatotoxicity occurs 72 to 96 hours after ingestion.[6]

9. **B. Assessment.** Salicylate poisoning initially will stimulate the respiratory center of the central nervous system. This manifests itself in an increased respiratory rate and causes respiratory alkalosis.[7]

10. **C. Intervention.** Salicylate poisoning is treated with gastric emptying, charcoal administration, and alkaline diuresis. Alkaline diuresis will increase the pH of the patient's urine and improve free salicylate excretion.[7]

11. **B. Analysis.** Salicylate poisoning may cause excessive fluid loss from nausea, vomiting, sweating, and hyperventilation, all of which can lead to dehydration.[7,9]

12. **C. Evaluation.** Bleeding problems may develop in severe salicylate poisoning. This occurs because of impaired platelet aggregation and decreased thrombin.[7]

13. **D. Assessment.** Because the most frequent cause of death in cyclic poisoning is related to cardiac toxicity, quickly placing the patient on the monitor and obtaining an ECG will help determine the amount of cyclic toxicity.[2]

14. **A. Intervention.** Cyclic poisoning can cause rapid changes in mental status and will easily place the patient at risk of vomiting and aspiration if the patient has been given anything orally. Cyclic antidepressants exert an

anticholinergic effect that may cause pills and pill fragments to remain in the stomach for a long period of time. Gastric lavage and then administration of charcoal will help ensure that the drug is removed from the patient's system.[2,11]

15. **C. Analysis.** The most appropriate nursing diagnosis would be C, because the toxic cardiac effects of cyclic antidepressant toxicity are lethal.[9]

16. **C. Evaluation.** Since the supply of norepinephrine is depleted by the body and the cyclic antidepressant is blocking the reuptake of norepinephrine, hypotension will result. It is important to recognize this toxic effect early so that appropriate intervention can be initiated.[2]

17. **B. Assessment.** Since hydrocarbon ingestion initially affects the respiratory system, the patient's respiratory system will need to be assessed. Included in this assessment should be the patient's normal respiratory rate and any indications of respiratory distress, including dyspnea, wheezes, stridor, hemoptysis, and cyanosis.[4]

18. **B. Intervention.** If the child has suffered pulmonary injury, supplemental oxygen will be needed.[4]

19. **D. Analysis.** One of the major complications with hydrocarbon ingestion is the potential for aspiration because of vomiting. The emergency nurse's plan of care needs to include interventions that will prevent any further injury to the pulmonary system from aspiration.[9]

20. **B. Evaluation.** An important role for the emergency nurse is teaching prevention. Obtaining information about the location of possible poisons and then teaching the child's parents how to prevent any further accidents could prevent a future tragedy.[9]

21. **A. Assessment.** The method of exposure needs to be considered, particularly in relation to insecticide poisoning. As noted in the history, the patient sprayed the insecticide all over himself in an enclosed place. He suffered not only inhalation exposure, but also dermal exposure. Therefore he will need to have his clothes removed and his skin cleansed with soap and water to remove any remaining insecticide.[8]

22. **C. Intervention.** Atropine is administered in doses of 1 to 5 mg and repeated every 15 minutes.[8]

23. **B. Analysis.** A suicidal patient is displaying ineffective coping. The patient has chosen behavior that is detrimental, and suicide precautions will need to be instituted while he is in the emergency department.[9]

24. **A. Evaluation.** Atropine will reverse the muscarinic effects of organophosphate poisoning, which include salivation, lacrimation, urinary and fecal incontinence, vomiting, miosis, bronchospasm, and bradycardia.[8,12]

REFERENCES

1. Litovitz TL, Schmitz B, Hilm K: 1989 Annual Report of the American Association of Poison Control Centers National Data Collection System, *Am J Emerg Med* 8:394-442, 1990.
2. Slovis C et al: Cyclic antidepressant OD: five classic patient types, *Emerg Med Rep* 8:113-120, 1987.
3. McNamara R et al: Efficacy of charcoal cathartic versus ipecac in reducing serum acetaminophen in a simulated overdose, *Ann Emerg Med* 18:934-938, 1989.
4. Ryals P: Hydrocarbons and petroleum distillates. In Noji EK, Kelen GD: editors: *Manual of toxicologic emergencies,* St Louis, 1989, Mosby–Year Book.
5. Stine R, Marcus R: Toxicologic emergencies. In Stine R, Marcus R, editors: *A practical approach to emergency medicine,* Boston, 1987, Little, Brown.
6. Riggs B: Acetaminophen. In Noji EK, Kelen GD, editors: *Manual of toxicologic emergencies,* St Louis, 1989, Mosby–Year Book.
7. Riggs B: Salicylates. In Noji EK, Kelen GD, editors: *Manual of toxicologic emergencies,* St Louis, 1989, Mosby–Year Book.
8. Haddad L, Winchester J: *Clinical management of poisoning and drug overdose,* Philadelphia, 1983, WB Saunders.
9. McFarland GK, McFarlane EA: *Nursing diagnosis and intervention: planning for patient care,* St Louis, 1989, Mosby–Year Book.
10. Wogan JM: Prevention of absorption. In Noji EK, Kelen GD, editors: *Manual of toxicologic emergencies,* St Louis, 1989, Mosby–Year Book.
11. Albertson TE et al: Superiority of activated charcoal in the treatment of acute toxic ingestions, *Ann Emerg Med* 18:56, 1989.
12. Sheehy SB: *Mosby's manual of emergency care,* ed 3, St Louis, 1990, Mosby–Year Book.

Chapter 20

Transportation and Stabilization

REVIEW OUTLINE

I. History of patient transport
   A. War transport
      1. European wars in the nineteenth century
      2. Civil war in the United States
      3. World War I
      4. World War II
      5. Korean War
      6. Vietnam War
   B. Civilian transport
      1. Hearse transport
      2. 1966 White Paper, "Trauma, the Neglected Disease of Modern Society"
      3. Department of Transportation Standards
      4. Emergency Medical Systems in the United States
   C. Air ambulance transport
      1. Balloons used in the nineteenth century
      2. Air ambulance service in the early 1900s
      3. First military transport in 1945
      4. Korean War
      5. Vietnam War
      6. First hospital-based helicopter program in 1972
II. Indications for transport
   A. Advanced care
      1. Level I or II trauma centers
      2. Pediatric care centers

3. Cardiac care centers
4. Neonatal care centers
5. Transplant centers
6. High-risk perinatal/neonatal centers
7. Reimplantation centers
8. Toxicological centers

B. Patient indications
1. Patients who require a certain type of nursing and/or medical expertise not available at the initial care facility
2. Patients who require diagnostic testing not available at the initial care facility
3. Patients whose condition may deteriorate and who require care not available at the initial care facility
4. Request by the patient's family that the patient be transferred to another facility

C. Methods for making transport decisions
1. Scoring systems
   a. Trauma score
   b. Pediatric trauma score
2. Local protocols
3. National standards
   a. Emergency Nurses Association (ENA)
   b. National Flight Nurses Association (NFNA)
   c. American College of Surgeons (ACS)

III. Consolidated Omnibus Budget Reconciliation Act (COBRA) (1986, 1989)
A. All hospitals must examine all patients who come to the emergency department and provide necessary medical care
B. Patients are not to be transferred until stabilized
C. The referring center must be able to document that the medical benefits for the patient are greater at the receiving center
D. The receiving facility must have available space and qualified personnel
E. Ambulances, fixed-wing aircraft, and helicopters must have appropriate equipment and personnel to perform the transfer

IV. Stabilization for transport
A. Airway stabilization
B. Ventilation
C. Circulation (cardiac monitor, control of bleeding)
D. Intravenous access
E. Assessment of vital signs
F. Neurological assessment

INTRODUCTION

In 1986 the Consolidated Omnibus Budget Reconciliation Act (COBRA) was passed, which, among other things, prohibits the "dumping" of patients by one hospital onto another. Several issues contributed to the development of this act, including an increase in the number of persons who do not have health insurance, the severity of the illnesses and injuries suffered by some people, and the cutting of health care budgets by both state and federal governments.

The COBRA law contains major implications for the practice of emergency nursing and medicine, including the following[1]:

- All hospitals must examine all patients who come to the emergency department and provide necessary medical care.
- Patients are not to be transferred until they are stabilized.
- It must be documented that the patient will receive better care at the receiving facility.
- The receiving facility must have available space and personnel to care for the patient.

Not all emergency departments and the facilities that they are a part of are able to take care of all the patients they are confronted with. The decision to transfer a patient should be based on many factors. Included in this decision-making process are the patient's need for additional expertise or additional diagnostic testing, possible deterioration in the patient's condition, and the family's request for transfer.

Hart et al.[2] listed the following reasons for transferring a patient:

- Serious injury to one or more organ systems
- Hypovolemic shock requiring more than one blood transfusion
- Spinal cord injuries
- Patients requiring advanced ventilatory support
- Head injuries with cerebrospinal fluid leakage, increased intracranial pressure (ICP), and a Glasgow Coma Scale rating of less than 9

Before patients are transferred, they need to be stabilized. Stabilization is based on securing the patient's airway, providing ventilation, and maintaining adequate circulation. In addition to meeting the physical needs of the patient, the emergency department doing the transferring needs to arrange for a receiving facility. Having policies, agreements, transfer forms, and specific procedures already established makes transferring the patient much easier for those involved.[3]

The final step in the process of stabilization and transportation is deciding what mode of transportation should be used to get a patient to the receiving facility. There are both advantages and disadvantages to ground and air ambulances. Advantages of ground ambulances include space and the ability to move in most types of weather. Disadvantages of ground transport include the length of time it may require to transport the patient, poor road conditions, and the lack of availability of personnel trained in advanced life support (ALS).[3]

The advantages of air transport include saving of time, crews with advanced skills and experience, and generally a smoother ride for the patient. Disadvantages of air transport include lack of available programs, weather restrictions, and limited space in which to provide patient care.[3]

REVIEW QUESTIONS
Pediatric Trauma

A 3-year-old child is brought to the emergency department after having been involved in a motor vehicle crash. Her injuries include a head injury with cerebrospinal fluid leakage, bruising in the left upper quadrant, and a fractured left femur.

Her vital signs are blood pressure, 80/50; pulse, 140; and respiratory rate, 8. A decision is made to transfer the child to the pediatric trauma center about 100 miles away.

1. In addition to documentation of the stabilization of the child's ABCs (airway, breathing, and circulation), what additional component of the initial assessment should be documented?
   0   A. The child's weight
   0   B. The neurological assessment
   0   C. The history of the accident
   0   D. The child's medical history

2. Based on the initial assessment of this child, the primary intervention the emergency nurse should prepare for is:
   0   A. Administering mannitol for ICP control
   0   B. Drawing blood for a type and crossmatch
   0   C. Intubation for airway management
   0   D. Applying MAST pants for hypotension

3. A tool that would be useful in the neurological evaluation of this patient is:
   0   A. The Modified Glasgow Coma Scale
   0   B. A cardiac monitor
   0   C. A Foley catheter
   0   D. Examination of deep tendon reflexes

4. The most appropriate nursing diagnosis for the emergency nursing care of this patient is:
   0   A. Fluid volume deficit, potential
   0   B. Infection, potential for
   0   C. Mobility, impaired physical
   0   D. Thought processes, altered

5. All of the following would indicate the need to transfer this patient *except:*
   0   A. Advanced diagnostic testing
   0   B. Nursing and medical expertise
   0   C. Lack of health insurance
   0   D. Serious injury to more than one organ system

Consolidated Omnibus Budget Reconciliation Act

A 55-year-old man is brought to the emergency department complaining of severe left-sided chest pain. The patient is placed on a cardiac monitor, and the emergency nurse runs an ECG. There is significant ST elevation noted in leads II, III, and aV_F. Because the patient may qualify for tissue plasminogen activator (t-PA) and it is not *available at this hospital, it has been decided that the patient should be transferred to another emergency department.*

6. The COBRA law would not be broken by transferring this patient because:
   - 0 A. The patient has good health insurance
   - 0 B. Initial care has not been given to this patient
   - 0 C. The transferring hospital cannot provide the care the patient needs
   - 0 D. There are several critical care unit beds available at the receiving facility

7. A helicopter program has been contacted to transport this patient to another emergency department. All of the following are advantages of helicopter transport for this patient *except:*
   - 0 A. A crew skilled in ALS
   - 0 B. Limited space in which to provide patient care
   - 0 C. Decreased time of transport
   - 0 D. A smoother trip for the patient

8. A disadvantage of using ground transport for this type of patient would be:
   - 0 A. Slower traveling time by ground than by air
   - 0 B. Total access to the patient
   - 0 C. More mobility of the crew within the vehicle
   - 0 D. Ability of the vehicle to stop quickly if needed to provide patient care

9. Of the following, the most important intervention in preparing this patient for transfer to another facility would be:
   - 0 A. Finding a facility willing to accept the patient
   - 0 B. Activating the transport system
   - 0 C. Initiating transport protocols
   - 0 D. Copying laboratory and x-ray findings

10. Of the following, the most appropriate nursing diagnosis for providing emergency nursing care when preparing this patient for transport would be:
    - 0 A. Injury, potential for
    - 0 B. Fluid volume excess
    - 0 C. Activity intolerance
    - 0 D. Cardiac output, decreased

ANSWERS

1. **B. Assessment.** Because of the child's severe head injury, the initial assessment should include an in-depth neurological assessment. The components of the neurological assessment should include the level of consciousness, pupillary response, motor response, sensory response, and vital signs.

2. **C. Intervention.** Because the child is hypoventilating—her respirations are 8—immediate control of the airway is indicated. Airway management may also help control any problems with ICP resulting from hyperventilation, as well as protect the child from aspiration.

3. **A. Assessment.** A Modified Glasgow Coma Scale has been developed for the pediatric patient. The differences between the pediatric and adult Glasgow Coma Scales include "Best Verbal Response" and "Best Motor Response."

4. **A. Analysis.** Because of the bruising on the child's upper left quadrant, the left fractured femur, and the initial vital signs, there is evidence that the child is at risk for the complications of hemorrhagic shock. The emergency nursing care for this patient would be organized within the nursing diagnosis fluid volume deficit, potential.

5. **C. Assessment.** One reason the COBRA law was drafted and passed in 1986 was to prevent hospitals from transferring or "dumping" patients for financial reasons. If a hospital is capable of providing needed patient services, it is obliged to do so. If this law is broken, the hospital may be fined $25,000 to $50,000 and lose its Medicare benefits. In addition, the injured party may be permitted to sue the hospital or anyone involved in his or her injury.[1]

6. **C. Intervention.** One of the major implications of the COBRA law is that patients should not be denied better medical care if it is available.[1]

7. **B. Intervention.** Using a helicopter to transfer this patient has the disadvantage of limited space in which to provide patient care.

8. **A. Intervention.** The major advantage air transportation has over ground transportation is the saving of time. It takes approximately one half to one third the time to travel by air than it does by ground. When the patient requires a certain procedure or medication wherein time is important, this disadvantage of being slower could influence patient outcome.[3]

9. **A. Intervention.** The first step in preparing the patient for transport would be to identify and contact a facility willing to receive the patient. A great deal of time and trouble can be saved if protocols and transfer agreements have already been established before any problems arise.[3] The

other issues are important, but not initially important if there is no place to send the patient.

10. **D. Analysis.** Since this patient's potential complications would most likely stem from his cardiac problems, the most appropriate nursing diagnosis would be cardiac output, decreased. Some of the defining characteristics of this nursing diagnosis are dysrhythmia and ECG changes. ECG changes have already been documented.

REFERENCES

1. Frew S, Roush W, La Greca K: COBRA: implications for emergency medicine, *Ann Emerg Med* 17:835-837, 1988.

2. Hart M et al: Air transport of the pediatric trauma patient, *Emerg Care Q* 3:21-26, 1987.

3. Rea R, editor: *Trauma nursing core course,* Chicago, 1987, Emergency Nurses Association.

Chapter 21 _____

Patient Care Management: Triage

REVIEW OUTLINE

I.   Definition of triage
    A. History of triage
       1. Military
       2. Civilian
    B. Types of triage
       1. Nursing
       2. Physician
       3. Paramedic, emergency medical technician (EMT)
       4. Disaster, multiple causality incident (MCI)
II. Components of triage
    A. ABCs (airway, breathing, circulation)
    B. Chief complaint
    C. History
    D. Classification
    E. Documentation
    F. Pediatric triage[1]
       1. Based on growth and development
       2. Use of history related by the parent or caregiver
       3. Based on assessment of the ABCs, recognizing the differences between the pediatric patient and the adult patient
       4. Use of tables that provide "normal" pediatric values, such as blood pressure, pulse, respirations, and weight
       5. General inspection of the child, looking for such things as rashes or signs of abuse or neglect
III. Rapid patient assessment
    A. Basic cardiac life support (BCLS)

    B. Advanced cardiac life support (ACLS)
    C. Pediatric advanced life support (PALS)
    D. Trauma nursing core curriculum (TNCC)
    E. Basic trauma life support (BTLS)
    F. Advanced trauma life support (ATLS)

IV. Chief complaint
    A. P = provocation
    B. Q = quality
    C. R = region and radiation
    D. S = severity of the problem
    E. T = time

V. History
    A. History related to the chief complaint
    B. Past medical history
    C. Allergies
    D. Cultural beliefs
    E. Family interaction

VI. Classification
    A. Emergent, urgent, nonurgent
    B. Immediate, expected, delayed care
    C. Acute, nonacute

VII. Documentation
    A. SOAP charting (subjective, objective, assessment, plan)
    B. Chief complaint
    C. History
    D. Brief physical assessment
    E. Family
    F. Allergies
    G. Tetanus status

VIII. Prehospital triage[2]
    A. Levels of care
        1. Level I (academic hospital)
        2. Level II (community hospital)
        3. Level III (rural hospital)
    B. Factors in patient assessment in prehospital triage
        1. Clinical status of the patient
        2. Nature and probable severity of the injury
        3. Type and availability of transportation
        4. Level of availability and accessibility of hospital care

IX. Nursing diagnoses

A. Airway clearance, ineffective
B. Breathing pattern, ineffective
C. Fluid volume deficit, potential
D. Injury, potential for
E. Knowledge deficit
F. Pain (acute); pain, chronic
G. Rape-trauma syndrome
H. Spiritual distress (distress of the human spirit)
I. Tissue perfusion, altered

INTRODUCTION

The word *triage* has its origin from the French, meaning "to pick, sort, select, or choose." The current use of *triage* in the emergency department is "to sort out" those in need of emergency services first. The concept of medical triage developed during battle; Napoleon's surgeon developed a system that "sorted out" the wounded on the battlefield. The most critically injured were transported first. Florence Nightingale, using her now-famous lamp, went out during the night after battles during the Crimean War to "sort out" the remaining soldiers and offer them care.[2]

At the end of the nineteenth century, the English introduced the use of causality and clearing stations where injuries were identified and first aid was initiated; based on their injuries, patients were then sent to an appropriate place for further treatment.[2]

During World War II and the Korean War, primary triage of the injured occurred on the battlefield, with secondary triage occurring at the battalion station and the final destination being a MASH unit.[2,3]

The introduction of helicopter transport of the injured from the battlefield helped to increase the speed at which victims were triaged and transported for care. Many causalities could be removed at the same time. Triage was done before and after air evacuation.

Civilian triage within hospitals formally began in the 1960s. Triage was initially done by physicians, but nurses quickly assumed primary triage responsibilities.[2,3]

The goals of triage include early patient assessment, brief overall assessment, determination of urgency need, documentation of findings during patient assessment, control of patient flow through the emergency department, assignment of patients to the appropriate care area, initiation of diagnostic measures, initiation of therapeutic interventions, infection control, promotion of good public relations, and health education for patients and families.[3] The goals and their implementation vary from emergency department to emergency department.

Triaging in the emergency department is based on both art and science. Experience, as well as the science of nursing and medicine, helps the emergency nurse in making assessment decisions. The *Journal of Emergency Nursing* contains a section entitled "Triage Decisions," which provides case studies about specific patient problems that may be seen in the emergency department. These can provide an excellent review for the nurse studying for the Certification in Emergency Nursing (CEN) examination.

REVIEW QUESTIONS

Three patients come to the triage nurse at once. The first patient is a 48-year-old man complaining of left-sided chest pain radiating down his left arm. He is awake, diaphoretic, and pale. The second patient is a 3-year-old boy who is drooling and pale, and who can only breathe sitting straight up on his mother's lap. The third patient has sustained a laceration on his right hand. He currently has a dressing in place, and bright red blood is noted on the dressing. His vital signs are a blood pressure of 100/70 and a pulse of 100.

1. Which patient should be taken into the emergency department first?
   - 0   A. The patient with the chest pain
   - 0   B. The child who is drooling
   - 0   C. The patient with the laceration
   - 0   D. Any patient who is bleeding

2. The triage nurse suspects that the child may have epiglottitis; what care should be provided in the triage area?
   - 0   A. Immediately remove the child from his mother
   - 0   B. Take an oral temperature
   - 0   C. Leave the child in his most comfortable position
   - 0   D. Immediately start an intraosseous infusion

3. The triage nurse should base the initial care of this patient on which of the following nursing diagnoses?
   - 0   A. Self-care deficit, feeding
   - 0   B. Infection, potential for
   - 0   C. Airway clearance, ineffective
   - 0   D. Family processes, altered

4. Audit criteria for triage documentation for a patient with potential airway problems (as in this case) should include documentation of:
0   A.   Insurance coverage
0   B.   The IV site and catheter size
0   C.   Chest x-ray results
0   D.   The patient's respiratory rate and effort

An 18-year-old man comes to the triage area complaining of upper body weakness, as well as numbness and tingling in both hands. The patient states that he was involved in a fight the previous night and that his head was shoved between his legs.

The patient is alert and oriented, vital signs are blood pressure, 110/70; pulse, 64; respiratory rate, 18; and temperature, 99° F. His pupils are equal and reactive. He is unable to keep his arms extended for longer than 5 seconds, and he cannot make a fist.

5. The triage classification for this patient would be:
0   A.   Delayed care
0   B.   Emergent
0   C.   Urgent
0   D.   Nonurgent

6. The initial care provided by the triage nurse should include application of:
0   A.   Heat to the patient's neck
0   B.   Ice to the patient's neck
0   C.   A cervical collar
0   D.   Ace wraps to the patient's hands

7. Of the following, which nursing diagnosis would be most appropriate for the care of this patient?
0   A.   Injury, potential for; trauma, potential for
0   B.   Fluid volume deficit, potential
0   C.   Hyperthermia
0   D.   Infection, potential for

8. Audit criteria for this patient (or any patient complaining of neurological trauma) should include documentation of:
0   A.   Breath sounds
0   B.   Peripheral pulses
0   C.   Romberg's test
0   D.   Pupillary response

An 83-year-old man is brought to the triage nurse by his granddaughter. She states that he has taken 25 tablets of Elavil, 50 mg. His wife recently died, and he is suffering from prostate cancer.

The patient states that he has a "living will" and has the right to die. He is refusing to allow the triage nurse to assess him.

9. Which of the following would be an appropriate action for the triage nurse to take?
    - 0   A. Allow the patient to leave
    - 0   B. Ask the granddaughter to leave
    - 0   C. Explain to the patient why he must stay
    - 0   D. Have the patient arrested

• • •

10. All of the following would be emergent conditions *except:*
    - 0   A. Obvious fractures with vascular compromise
    - 0   B. Hemorrhage from a wound
    - 0   C. Cardiopulmonary arrest
    - 0   D. Respiratory distress

11. Which of the following heart rates would alert the triage nurse to a problem in an infant?
    - 0   A. 120 beats per minute
    - 0   B. 160 beats per minute
    - 0   C. 130 beats per minute
    - 0   D. 220 beats per minute

12. The goals of triage include all of the following *except:*
    - 0   A. Control of patient flow through the emergency department
    - 0   B. Assignment of patients to appropriate care areas within the emergency department
    - 0   C. Performing and documenting a secondary survey on all patients who come to triage
    - 0   D. Determination of the urgency of the patient's condition

ANSWERS

1. **B. Assessment.** Based on rapid patient assessment using both basic and advanced life support principles (airway, breathing, circulation, neurological deficit, exposure [ABCDE], and history), the patient having airway

difficulties should be taken into the emergency department first. A child who is drooling and only able to breathe comfortably sitting straight up may have epiglottitis and is at great risk of completely obstructing his airway.[1-3]

2. **C. Intervention.** Since the child is currently able to comfortably maintain his airway, the triage nurse should leave the child in the position in which he is most comfortable. By removing him from his mother or performing any unnecessary procedures, the nurse may cause the child to become agitated and obstruct his airway.[1-3]

3. **C. Analysis.** Since the patient is having airway difficulties, airway clearance, ineffective, should be the initial nursing diagnosis on which the emergency nurse bases care. Defining characteristics of this nursing diagnosis include abnormal breath sounds, cyanosis, tachypnea, and dyspnea.[4]

4. **D. Evaluation.** The patient's respiratory rate is an important piece of information for the patient who is having respiratory difficulties and should be documented on the triage record. One of the responsibilities of the triage nurse is to sort out patients and determine the need for emergency services. The patient's vital signs provide the emergency nurse with observed information about the patient's cardiopulmonary status.[3]

5. **B. Assessment.** Based on rapid patient assessment using ABCDE, this patient would be an emergent patient. He has signs and symptoms of a neurological deficit that could place him at risk for additional complications related to injury of the cervical spine.[1]

6. **C. Intervention.** One of the goals of triage is the initiation of therapeutic interventions. Because this patient may have suffered a cervical spine injury, the initial care of this patient should include immobilization of the cervical spine.[1,3]

7. **A. Analysis.** The initial assessment of the patient demonstrates that he is currently in no acute distress, but because of his mechanism of injury and symptoms is at great risk for additional injury. Defining characteristics of this nursing diagnosis are divided into host factors such as sensory or motor deficits, tissue hypoxia, and cognitive impairment; agent factors such as chemical and mechanical energy; and environmental factors such as unsafe design, unsafe mode of transportation, and presence of pollutants.[4]

8. **D. Evaluation.** Documentation of a neurological examination includes the level of consciousness, pupillary response, motor response, sensory response, and vital signs.

9. **C. Intervention.** The triage nurse should first try to explain to the patient that a living will does not allow the patient to deliberately harm himself. Rather, the living will allows the patient to decide whether or not medical

or nursing care should be given if the patient is dying from natural causes. The emergency department is obligated to treat the patient.[5]

10. **A. Assessment.** One method of triage classification is the use of specific patient designations: emergent, urgent, and nonurgent. Emergent patients include those with cardiopulmonary arrest, chest pain indicative of a myocardial infarction, respiratory distress, severe trauma, and attempted suicide. Urgent patients include those with obvious fractures with vascular compromise, abdominal pain of less than 36 hours' duration, sudden headaches, vomiting, and jaundice. Nonurgent patients include those with sprains, minor burns, and closed fractures.[6]

11. **D. Assessment.** The normal infant's heart rate will range from 120 to 160 (newborn to 1 year of age). A heart rate greater than 200 is an indication of some type of problem.[7]

12. **C. Intervention.** Performing and documenting a secondary survey on all patients who come to triage is an unrealistic goal. The primary goal of triage is to recognize the ill or injured patient who requires treatment in a timely manner. Triage areas are generally not set up to perform an adequate secondary assessment.[7]

REFERENCES

1. Thomas D: The ABCs of pediatric triage, *JEN* 14:154-159, 1988.
2. Champion H: Prehospital triage. In *Trauma care systems,* Rockville, Md, 1986, Aspen.
3. Rund DA, Rausch TS: *Triage,* St Louis, 1981, Mosby–Year Book.
4. McFarland GK, McFarlane EA: *Nursing diagnosis and intervention: planning for patient care,* St Louis, 1989, Mosby–Year Book.
5. Cole J, Plantz S: *Emergency medicine: self-assessment and review,* New York, 1990, McGraw-Hill.
6. Sheehy SB, Barber J: *Emergency nursing: principles and practice,* ed 2, St Louis, 1985, Mosby–Year Book.
7. Sheehy SB: *Mosby's manual of emergency care,* ed 3, St Louis, 1990, Mosby–Year Book.

Chapter 22
Research

REVIEW OUTLINE

I. Research process
    A. Identification of the research question or problem
        1. From practice
        2. Duplication of previous study
        3. Case study
        4. Quality assurance
        5. Patient follow-ups
    B. Review of the literature
    C. Theoretical framework
    D. Defining research variables or definition of terms
    E. Hypothesis or research questions
    F. Research design
        1. Experimental
        2. Quasi-experimental
        3. Descriptive
        4. Exploratory
        5. Methodological
    G. Measurement of the variables
    H. Data collection
    I. Data analysis
    J. Interpretation of the results
    K. Communication of the results
II. Clinical problem solving

INTRODUCTION

Research and clinical problem solving provide methods of discovering and evaluating new ideas (knowledge) in the practice of emergency nursing. Examples of clinical problem solving include quality assurance projects, case studies and conferences, and chart auditing.

The research process is composed of multiple steps, including identification of the problem, review of the literature, development of a theoretical framework, definition of research variables, hypothesis formation or formation of research questions, selection of a research design, sample selection, measurement of variables, collection of the data, data analysis, interpretation of the results, and communication of the research findings.[1-3]

REVIEW QUESTIONS

1. When deciding which IV insertion technique may save time when used in the emergency department, the emergency nurse may use which of the following?
   - 0   A. Chart audits
   - 0   B. Current studies
   - 0   C. Case studies
   - 0   D. All of the above

2. An important role the emergency nurse plays in the research even if he or she is not conducting the study is:
   - 0   A. Collection of data
   - 0   B. Interpretation of data
   - 0   C. Protection of patients' rights
   - 0   D. Deciding the study design

3. The first step in the research process is:
   - 0   A. Obtaining patient consent
   - 0   B. Identifying the problem or question
   - 0   C. Reviewing the current literature
   - 0   D. Selecting a research design

4. The following are examples of research instruments *except:*
   - 0   A. Review of the literature
   - 0   B. Pulse oximeter

0   C. Focused interviews
0   D. Questionnaires

5. Clinical problem solving is similar to the research process in all of the following ways *except:*
    0   A. Clinical problem solving tries to provide solutions to a problem
    0   B. Clinical problem solving looks at problems in the clinical setting
    0   C. Clinical problem solving is theory based
    0   D. Clinical problem solving uses statistics in data analysis

ANSWERS

1. **D.** All of these methods would serve to help the emergency nurse solve this particular problem. A review of the literature may reveal that a study has already been conducted that provides the information the emergency nurse is seeking.
2. **C.** One of the most important roles that the emergency nurse plays in the research process—whether or not he or she is conducting the study— is the assurance of the protection of human subjects. Emergency department patients are a very vulnerable group of people. The emergency nurse may need to act as an advocate not only to be sure that the patient understands the study, but also to support patients if they choose not to participate.[1]
3. **B.** The first step in the research process is identifying the research problem or formulating the research question. Before one can begin the research process, one needs to first identify what one is going to study. Important delineations to make when identifying a nursing research problem or question include whether the problem or question will add to the body of nursing knowledge, will improve nursing practice, or will provide solutions that will explain, describe, identify, or predict behavior.
4. **A.** Review of the literature is a step in the research process. The other answers provide examples of instruments the emergency nurse may use to gather data about a research problem in the emergency department.
5. **C.** Clinical problem solving and the research process are similar in some ways and very different in others. One of the major differences between the two is that clinical problem solving is not theory based. Both try to solve clinical problems, and both may use some type of statistics to evaluate the

data. However, the research process uses a theoretical framework for organization of the study and as the foundation on which to generate more nursing knowledge based on previous knowledge.[2]

REFERENCES

1. Polit D, Hungler B: *Nursing research,* Philadelphia, 1987, JB Lippincott.
2. Mateo MA, Kirchoff KT: *Conducting and using nursing research in the clinical setting,* Baltimore, 1991, Williams & Wilkins.
3. Burns N, Grove SK: *The practice of nursing research: conduct, critique and utilization,* Philadelphia, 1987, WB Saunders.

Chapter 23

Patient Education and Discharge Planning

REVIEW OUTLINE

I. Teaching/learning process
   A. Identification of learning needs
   B. Assessment of the learner
      1. Readiness to learn
      2. Present anxiety level
      3. Capability to learn
      4. Motivation
   C. Establishment of goals
   D. Selection of teaching methods
      1. Verbal
      2. Written
         a. Home care instruction sheets
         b. Patient-specific instructions
      3. Visual aids
      4. Question-and-answer session
      5. Return demonstration
   E. Provision of adequate time
II. Content
   A. Disease, disorder, or injury
      1. Causes
      2. Predisposing and precipitating factors
      3. Expected course
      4. Plan of care
   B. Diagnostic test or procedure
      1. Equipment

2. Activity
3. Outcome
C. Discharge, home care
   1. Equipment and supplies needed
   2. Step-by-step procedure
   3. Specifics regarding medications
   4. Pertinent observations
   5. Appropriate follow-up
   6. Changes requiring immediate intervention
   7. Community resource referral, if indicated
D. Prevention
   1. Prevention of recurrence
   2. Prevention of infection
   3. General hygiene
III. Evaluation, documentation

INTRODUCTION

An important responsibility of the emergency nurse is that of patient education. The nurse assumes the role of health teacher in preparing each patient and/or significant other to assume patient care on leaving the emergency department. This is a vital nursing task, essential to the practice of emergency nursing.

One must be familiar with the process of teaching and use the time available to prepare the patient for discharge. Ideally, patient teaching begins at the first nurse-patient encounter and continues throughout the patient's stay. Saving all the information until actual discharge can be overwhelming to both patient and nurse. It is much more effective to do nursing care teaching in parts during the patient's stay so that the patient has time to digest information and ask questions. Discharge is best used as a time of summary and return verbalization of instructions by the patient to ensure understanding. There are a number of obstacles to overcome in preparing patients to successfully care for themselves. The stress of a busy, noisy department can increase the anxiety already felt by the patient, and a high anxiety level clouds the learning process. The nurse helps to decrease this stress through both verbal and nonverbal means. Simple acts such as explaining tests and procedures in understandable terms and listening carefully to what the patient has to say can allay anxiety. Likewise, nonverbal communication in facial expression, touch, and body language is effective.[1]

The vast array of health problems encountered in the emergency setting makes it imperative for the nurse to have a broad range of teaching skills. Whereas the obstetrical nurse or orthopedic nurse is usually dealing with a single issue, the emergency nurse must be able to prepare patients with a variety of health problems for home care.[1]

Issues of importance to be taught during the patient's emergency visit include cause and prevention of the injury or illness and possible complications. Lengthy explanations are not necessary; simple descriptions usually suffice. The patient who understands something about what has happened is more likely to be compliant with treatment and more likely to know how to work toward prevention of a similar episode in the future. This information also assists the patient in recognizing any complications that may arise and in seeking further intervention as necessary.

Obviously, the patient must learn about nursing care measures specific to his or her problem. Discharge instructions given by the physician are not sufficient. Nursing care is best taught by nurses. Such items as wound care, fever control, and walking with crutches are examples of the myriad of things patients must understand in order to get well at home. Also, the nurse must have learned enough about the patient's home situation to help the patient adapt care routines to his or her needs. For example, does the patient with a leg cast have stairs that must be traveled at home? Does the mother of a febrile child have a thermometer, and does she know how to use it? These are nursing problems that need to be solved before the patient leaves the emergency department.

Another educational need the nurse meets in preparing the patient for discharge concerns prescribed medications. It is important that the patient understand the expected actions and possible side effects, as well as specifics for taking or using the medication. Reviewing with the patient how to use a suppository or the importance of taking a particular drug with food can ensure compliance.

Finally, documentation of patient education must be recorded. Many institutions have standardized care instructions available for specific uses, such as wound care and head injury observation. Notation that these are given to the patient is made. Instructions specific to the individual are written, ideally with a duplicate for the patient to take home. Again, it is important that these instructions be in terms the patient can understand, and, of course, they must be legible. The nurse notes on the patient's records who received the instuctions and that the receiver verbalized understanding. The chart should be signed by the patient or significant other, verifying this.

Patient teaching in the emergency setting is essential to good care. Patients who leave the emergency department with an adequate understanding of how to care for their problem at home are more likely to recover without complications. Good discharge information often prevents unnecessary return visits and time-consuming phone calls back to the facility. Patient satisfaction is enhanced when educational needs are met.

REVIEW QUESTIONS

1. An 8-month-old girl is being discharged from the emergency department with bilateral otitis media. In addition to instructions for fever control and medication administration, the nurse tells the mother to:
   0   A. Weigh the baby daily
   0   B. Isolate the baby from other children until the fever is gone
   0   C. Discontinue formula, substituting clear liquids
   0   D. Avoid putting the baby to bed with a bottle

2. Antibiotics are prescribed for this infant. It is important for the nurse to include in her teaching all of the following *except:*
   0   A. Give the antibiotic until it is gone
   0   B. If the baby vomits her medicine, wait 30 minutes and repeat
   0   C. Discontinue the medication and notify the physician if the baby is not better in 3 days
   0   D. Continue fever control measures in addition to giving the antibiotic

3. In reviewing fever control measures with the parent, the nurse learns that the parent has no acetaminophen but does have baby aspirin. Based on the baby's age and weight of 19 pounds, the appropriate dose of aspirin is:
   0 · A. Half a baby aspirin every 4 hours
   0   B. Half a baby aspirin every 6 hours
   0   C. One baby aspirin every 6 hours
   0   D. Aspirin is not appropriate for this patient

4. A 32-year-old man is being discharged from the emergency department with a diagnosis of left corneal abrasion sustained at work. He has a patch in place and has been given antibiotic ointment to use. The most important teaching to be done for this patient would be:
   0   A. Stressing the importance of not driving or operating other machinery while wearing the patch
   0   B. Teaching him how to apply the ointment

0 C. Reminding him how long the patch is to be worn

0 D. Stressing the importance of wearing goggles at work to prevent recurrence of this injury

5. A 10-year-old boy is being discharged from the emergency department with a right forearm fracture sustained in a fall. He has a long arm plaster cast in place. An important skill to teach his parent would be:

0 A. How to get a pullover shirt on and off

0 B. How to do circulation checks

0 C. How to take care of itching under the cast

0 D. How to elevate the child's arm

6. Another bit of advice pertinent for this patient would be:

0 A. How to trim excess padding from around the cast

0 B. To avoid striking the cast against anything

0 C. How to dry the cast if it gets wet

0 D. That writing on the cast can begin on arrival home

7. A 42-year-old man is being discharged from the emergency department with a diagnosis of low back strain after lifting a refrigerator. His discharge instructions are based on which of the following nursing diagnoses?

0 A. Pain

0 B. Activity intolerance

0 C. Mobility, impaired physical

0 D. All of the above

8. The physician has prescribed cyclobenzaprine hydrochloride (a muscle relaxant) and ibuprofen for this patient. Specific nursing instructions regarding these medications include all of the following *except:*

0 A. Activity is permitted as tolerated while the patient is taking these medications

0 B. Ibuprofen should be taken with food or milk

0 C. Cyclobenzaprine hydrochloride may cause drowsiness

0 D. Bed rest will hasten recovery

9. A 52-year-old woman has been treated in the emergency department for stable angina and is ready for discharge with sublingual nitroglycerin. The most important instruction she receives is:

0 A. How to take nitroglycerin

   0   B. How to restrict activity
   0   C. When to follow up with her private physician
   0   D. To seek medical attention immediately if pain persists after taking nitroglycerin

10. Side effects of nitroglycerin to be reviewed with this patient include:
   0   A. Dizziness, transient headache, blurred vision, flushing
   0   B. Dizziness, lightheadedness, transient headache, flushing
   0   C. Lightheadedness, persistent headache, blurred vision, rash
   0   D. Dizziness, fainting, transient headache, rash

ANSWERS

1. **D. Intervention.** Babies who are routinely put to bed with a bottle are more prone to recurrent bouts of otitis media. They often fall asleep in the act of sucking, which increases pressure in the eustachian tubes, inhibiting free drainage and providing a good place for infection to begin. Parents should be encouraged to hold the baby until the bottle is finished. This will prevent prolonged negative pressure in the eustachian tubes, as well as promote bonding between parent and infant.

2. **C. Intervention.** Good patient/family teaching for anyone discharged while taking antibiotics is essential. The patient, or in this case the parent, needs to understand that the medication prescribed will help the infection but does not work immediately, and that the full course is required. It should be stressed that antibiotics do not reduce fever; standard fever control is needed. It is not uncommon to have some vomiting with otitis media. Persistent vomiting, though, is cause for concern. Antibiotics should not be discontinued without physician consultation.

3. **D. Intervention.** The use of aspirin for fever control in infants and children has been linked to the development of Reye's syndrome and is therefore contraindicated. Acetaminophen will reduce fever without harmful side effects in appropriate dosage. Methods for obtaining this drug, preferably in elixir form, should be explored with the mother before she goes home.

4. **A. Intervention.** When one eye is patched, depth perception is severely altered. To prevent injury to himself and others, the patient should avoid activity wherein intact vision is crucial to safety.

5. **B. Intervention.** All of these items would contribute to the patient's comfort and well-being at home. However, recognizing excessive swelling within the cast by means of altered circulation checks is essential. The

capillary refill test is a simple procedure that is taught to all patients who are discharged with any type of circumferential dressing in place.

6. **B. Intervention.** A plaster cast is to be kept dry and all padding left as is. A 24-hour drying time is needed, and during that time handling of the cast should be careful and minimal; therefore writing on it should be deferred until after that time. This patient's age, sex, and mechanism of injury should alert the nurse to the need to stress that the cast is not to be used as a weapon to strike objects or other people. Active children and young men seem prone to this activity and need to be discouraged from it. On impact, the cast may be damaged, causing further damage to the already injured area. Of course, the possibility of harm to other people or objects is obvious.

7. **D. Analysis.** This patient's instructions will include use of prescribed medications and nursing comfort measures to be followed at home, as well as prevention of future similar injury. In discussing each of these points with the patient, the nurse is imparting knowledge specific to him and his current problem.

8. **A. Intervention.** Pain control and muscle relaxation are the goals of these medications and will be enhanced with bed rest. Strained muscles heal more quickly with rest, and medication cannot be considered a substitute.

9. **D. Intervention.** Pain not relieved with rest and three successive nitroglycerin tablets may well herald a serious myocardial event. A patient with known stable angina should be reminded when and how to seek help.

10. **B. Evaluation.** The vasodilating effects of this drug are responsible for the transient dizziness, lightheadedness, headache, and flushing of the face and neck that some people experience.[2] The duration of action with sublingual nitroglycerin is very short; therefore any persistent events such as blurred vision, fainting, rash, or prolonged headache should be reported to the physician.

REFERENCES

1. Sheehy SB, Barber J: *Emergency nursing: principles and practice,* ed 2, St Louis, 1985, Mosby–Year Book.

2. Karch A, Boyd E: *Handbook of drugs,* Philadelphia, 1989, JB Lippincott.

ADDITIONAL READING

1. Rea R et al: *Emergency nursing core curriculum,* ed 3, Philadelphia, 1987, WB Saunders.

Chapter 24

Organization and Personnel Management

REVIEW OUTLINE

I. Medicolegal aspects of emergency nursing
   A. General overview
      1. Hospital's duty to provide care
         a. Wilmington General Hospital vs. Manlove (1961): the hospital's duty to provide care outweighs the hospital's internal policies
         b. Hill-Burton Act (1946): if the hospital receives federal funds under this act, it must provide care regardless of the patient's ability to pay or the nature of the presenting complaint
      2. Nurse's duty to provide care
         a. State nurse practice act: duty and responsibilities defined
         b. Hospital employment policies: obligation to follow directions and fulfill duties
      3. Types of law
         a. Constitutional: determines the validity of both the statutory decision and the case law within the provisions of the fourth, fifth, and fourteenth constitutional amendments
         b. Statutory: law enacted by a legislative body
         c. Regulatory: regulations developed by an official under empowerment by statutory law
         d. Case: interpretation by the courts on statutes, administrative rules, and common law
         e. Contract: written, oral, or implied agreement between parties
      4. General legal terms, concepts
         a. Standards of care
            (1) Provide guidelines

(2) ORPP: ordinary, reasonable, prudent person with like or similar training in like or similar circumstances

b. Negligence: omission or commission of an act that should or should not have been performed, coupled with unreasonableness and/or imprudence on the part of the doer

(1) Standard

(2) Deviation from standard

(3) Elements of negligence

    a. Duty

    b. Breach of contract

    c. Proximate cause

    d. Damage or injury

c. Malpractice: negligence on the part of a professional when his or her misconduct, lack of skill, omission, or misjudgment in the commission of duty causes harm to the person or property of the recipient of services

d. Tort: unintentional negligent act on the person of another that results in injury to that person

5. Assault: threat to do harm to another without the actual performance of that threatened harm

6. Battery: actual touching of another person without the person's consent

7. False imprisonment: restrictions of a person's right to freedom of movement

8. Good Samaritan law

B. Consent to treatment

1. Types of consent

    a. Informed express consent

      (1) Voluntary

      (2) Informed

    b. Implied

    c. Involuntary

    d. Minor's consent

      (1) Emancipated minor

      (2) Nonemancipated minor

2. Refusal of treatment, AMA (against medical advice) situation

C. Reportable situations

1. Reporting requirements

2. Reportable events

D. Emergency department record
1. Joint Commission on Accreditation of Health Organizations (JCAHO) requirements
2. Documentation requirements
3. Confidentiality
4. Release of information
   a. Privacy act
   b. Rights of press
   c. Hospital policy
5. Patient transfers: Consolidated Omnibus Budget Reconciliation Act (COBRA)
6. Patient discharge and instructions
7. Chain-of-evidence collection
E. Specific emergency situations
1. Triage guidelines
   a. Hospital policy
   b. State law
   c. Nurse practice act
2. Telephone advice
   a. Develop and follow policies and procedures
   b. Document
3. Restraining of patients
   a. Out-of-control behavior
   b. Danger to self or others
   c. Nursing considerations
4. Psychiatric patients
   a. Assess danger to self or others
   b. Holds
5. Blood alcohol/drug level sampling
   a. Hospital policy
   b. State law
   c. Medical purposes vs. police request
II. Professional issues in emergency nursing
A. Practice
1. Standards of emergency practice
2. Job performance and competency skills
3. Extended practice roles
B. Education
1. Nurse's role in education of self, peers, and/or patients

2. Continuing education
3. Competency skills
4. Certification

C. Research
    1. Components of the research process
        a. Identification of the problem or question
        b. Review of the literature
        c. Research design
        d. Data collection
        e. Instruments
        f. Data analysis
        g. Implications for emergency nursing practice
    2. Ethics of research in the emergency department
        a. Rights of human subjects
        b. Availability of research protocols
        c. Emergency nursing's role in research

D. Leadership, management, personnel management
    1. Roles and responsibilities
    2. Resource management
        a. Personnel
            (1) Staffing, scheduling
            (2) Hiring, disciplining
            (3) Supplies, equipment
        b. Budgeting
            (1) Capital budget
            (2) Operating budget
            (3) Revenue projections
    3. Education of staff
        a. Comprehensive orientation
        b. Planned formal training programs
        c. Departmental training programs
        d. Competency skills testing and proof of annual review
    4. JCAHO
        a. Fire
        b. Safety
        c. Infection control
        d. Other requirements
    5. Regulatory requirements
        a. Medicaid
        b. Medicare

      c. Health Care Financing Administration (HCFA)

      d. JCAHO

      e. Preferred provider organizations (PPOs)

      f. Health maintenance organizations (HMOs)

      g. Hill-Burton Act

   6. Quality assurance

      a. Ten-step process

      b. Systematic, planned, ongoing, integrated

   7. Budgeting

      a. Operational

      b. Capital

      c. Revenue

   8. Strategic planning

      a. Vision for the future

      b. Staff involvement

   9. Marketing

      a. Internal

      b. External

      c. Competition

      d. Consumer needs

III. Organization of the emergency department

  A. JCAHO standards: overview of content

    1. Department has a well-developed plan for emergency care for levels I through IV, based on community needs and the defined capability of the hospital

    2. Department is properly directed and staffed according to the nature and extent of the health care needs anticipated and the scope of services offered

    3. Department is appropriately integrated with other departments

    4. Personnel are prepared for job responsibilities through appropriate training and educational programs

    5. There are written policies and procedures for the scope and conduct of patient care to be provided

    6. Department is designed and equipped to facilitate the safe and effective care of patients

    7. Medical records are appropriately maintained on all patients

    8. Department has established appropriate quality control mechanisms

    9. Quality and appropriateness of patient care provided are monitored and evaluated

  B. Regulatory mechanisms affecting provision of care and reimbursement

1. JCAHO
2. HCFA
3. Hill-Burton
4. Medicaid
5. Medicare
6. Federal and state legislation
7. PPOs, HMOs, etc.
8. Hospital policy

INTRODUCTION

The emergency department manager today is faced with many organizational and personnel management issues. While it is an exciting time, it is also one of constant change and competition. Consumer expectations, prospective payment, and various regulatory requirements have made the care of the emergency department patient very complex. A variety of financial and administrative issues regulate who is treated, how they are treated, what is done for specific patients, when they are treated, and whether they are seen in the emergency department or are referred to a variety of other settings (physician's office, clinic, etc.) for initial treatment and/or follow-up. These issues have made the marketing aspects of emergency department management essential to maintain financial viability and to comply with regulatory requirements.

This competitive arena has forced managers to look at financial issues from operational, strategic, and revenue standpoints. Managers must look at the best ways to use resources and contain costs while maintaining a happy, motivated staff who feel valued. At the same time, managers must maintain and/or improve the quality of patient care. "Doing more with less (or at least without adding more) and doing it better and faster" has become the standard slogan for managers in the 1990s. This has forced managers to seek greater involvement from staff and to keep them better informed of health care changes impacting emergency care. Nurses play a significant role in the financial success of the emergency department. They must be involved with containing costs and enhancing departmental profitability because they are the ones who must efficiently and knowledgeably manage their use of personnel and material resources on a daily basis. This calls for increased teamwork in the emergency care setting.

It is only through teamwork in the emergency department that the increasing needs of consumers can be consistently met. Consumers are better educated and sophisticated about health care issues, including costs, services, what they should expect, and what quality care means. They frequently search for the "best" place(s) to obtain health care and may not return to the same emergency department if they were dissatisfied with previous care or with the way they were treated.

The emergency department still serves as a clinic or replacement for the patient's personal physician, as well as a trauma center. Emergency services constitute the largest portion of hospital-based outpatient services.[1] The emergency department remains the entry point to the health care delivery system and serves as an interface between the hospital, emergency medical service (EMS) systems, and community referral agencies.

The proliferation of HMOs, PPOs, and other employee benefit plans has greatly affected the use of emergency departments. Obtaining approval prior to being seen in the emergency department to ensure payment has been implemented by many of these organizations. The intent of this practice is to discourage people from inappropriately using the emegency department, and although it has helped relieve some of the abuse or misuse of the emergency department, it has, at the same time, increased the number of phone calls made and created additional required paperwork and documentation for staff members. With these increasing demands being placed on emergency departments, many managers have focused closely on patient relations endeavors and on new ways to recruit and retain staff to deal efficiently and effectively with these issues.

Emergency department nurse managers are required to make provisions to assure staff competency. Nurses are required to possess skill levels enabling them to deal effectively with patients with more critical (acute) problems, as well as with critical care patients who are often held in the emergency department as a result of overcrowding. Emergency department nurses are required to prove their competency through annual competency skill checks. In addition, they must attend continuing education programs to obtain new knowledge and to remain confident, comfortable, and prepared. This also places additional financial demands on the departmental budget that the emergency department manager must remember when forecasting future budgets.

JCAHO has developed standards and criteria required to provide a safe, well-staffed, well-equipped department with competent personnel. (See the nine JCAHO standards in the Review Outline [Section III, A].)

The focus on ongoing monitoring and evaluation of information about important aspects of patient care remains a requirement of JCAHO. It also remains a "must" for emergency department managers if they are to truly keep in touch with patient care management issues and ensure quality care.

For the above reasons, budgeting, financial planning, and management are more important than ever. Operational, capital, and revenue budgets must be planned well and executed carefully. Strategic planning is a must for emergency department managers if they are to stay ahead of the game and remain financially viable in this competitive environment.

Care of the uninsured and underinsured remains a problem in the health care industry and in emergency departments, specifically. Although equal access to quality health care for all patients is essential, frequently the uninsured and underinsured patients find themselves without adequate access to health care or adequate care delivery. The Consolidated Omnibus Reconciliation Act (COBRA) of 1986 requires that all patients with emergency conditions and women in active labor be treated regardless of ability to pay for treatment rendered. This act requires any hospital receiving Medicare funds to evaluate all emergency patients to determine whether an emergency condition exists. If it does, the hospital must provide immediate and stabilizing care before transfer is considered.

The demands placed on emergency department managers are thus obvious and complex. These managers must ensure that (1) they remain current in the specialty, (2) appropriate policies and procedures are developed and continually revised, (3) appropriate measures are taken to provide a safe environment for staff members, (4) adequate numbers of qualified staff are available to provide care, (5) staff members remain competent, (6) and legal issues are addressed.

REVIEW QUESTIONS
The Patient Who Is Confused

A 75-year-old man with a history of intermittent confusion and disorientation is brought to the emergency department. The nursing home record confirms the report given by EMS personnel that the patient has wandered about the nursing home during periods of confusion and disorientation and fallen without injury on more than one occasion. On admission, the patient is alert, oriented, and joking with the nurse about how young he feels. Fifteen minutes later, he becomes confused and disoriented, trying to get out of bed to turn on the radio.

1. The nursing diagnosis for this patient that calls for immediate nursing intervention is:
   - 0   A. Thought processes, altered
   - 0   B. Injury, potential for
   - 0   C. Mobility, impaired physical
   - 0   D. Infection, potential for

2. Nursing interventions for this patient should include:
- 0   A.   Side rails and jacket restraint
- 0   B.   Side rails, restraints, and sedation
- 0   C.   Four-point leather restraints
- 0   D.   Watching the patient closely without restraint

3. The nurse caring for this patient fails to put up one of the side rails and does not place the patient in a restraint device. The patient subsequently falls out of bed. X-ray studies reveal that the patient has sustained a fractured hip and wrist. If the family decides to sue this nurse, they will probably file suit for:
- 0   A.   Negligence
- 0   B.   Malpractice
- 0   C.   Battery
- 0   D.   Felony

Personnel Management

A 32-year-old female nurse is brought into the emergency department (where she works) under CPR following an automobile accident. She subsequently dies. The staff are upset and at a loss because they were unable to resuscitate her.

4. The *least* helpful thing the emergency department manager could do to alleviate the staff's distress would be to:
- 0   A.   Provide coverage for them so that they could all leave
- 0   B.   Call the chaplain to talk with them
- 0   C.   Offer critical incident stress debriefing (CISD) to encourage them to talk about their feelings
- 0   D.   Make sure they finished charting and then kept busy with other patients

5. The *most* helpful action the emergency department manager could take to assist with dealing with all involved staff in this situation would be to:
- 0   A.   Provide coverage for them so that they could all leave
- 0   B.   Call the chaplain to talk with them
- 0   C.   Offer critical incident stress debriefing (CISD) to encourage them to talk about their feelings
- 0   D.   Ask the attending physician to prescribe tranquilizers

JCAHO Standards

6. One of the JCAHO standards requires that personnel be prepared for their emergency care responsibilities through appropriate training and educational programs. This is accomplished, as required, by all of the following *except:*

   0 A. Detailed orientation and ongoing inservice educational programs

   0 B. Documented annual review of competency skills

   0 C. Evidence of participation in planned formal training programs

   0 D. Orientation on beginning employment only

Research

7. On entering the trauma room, the emergency nurse finds the surgical resident beginning to start a research protocol drug on the patient who has just arrived. The patient is alert and oriented. What should the emergency nurse's first reaction be?

   0 A. To ask the resident if the patient has signed the required research consent

   0 B. To not worry about bothering the patient with paperwork, since the patient is a trauma patient

   0 C. To ask the patient if he knows the resident is administering an investigational drug to him

   0 D. To notify the resident's superior

Legal Issues

8. A 15-year-old boy is brought to the emergency department by his 18-year-old sister. He is complaining of flulike symptoms. Permission to treat should be received from the:

   0 A. Patient's parents

   0 B. Patient's sister

   0 C. Hospital administrator

   0 D. Local court system

9. A 46-year-old woman is brought into the emergency department. She has the smell of alcohol on her breath. On transfer to the treatment stretcher, she becomes violent, cursing at staff and attempting to hit anyone nearby. The first priority of the emergency department nurse would be to:

   0 A. Call security and have the patient taken to jail

   0 B. Try to calm the patient by establishing rapport

   0 C. Protect the patient, family, and staff from physical harm

   0 D. Prepare the patient for transfer to a psychiatric facility

10. A 24-year-old woman known to have diabetes passes out at work and hits her head. She is incoherent for a few seconds after she is awakened from the incident and is brought to the emergency department. After the patient is seen by the nurse and physician, blood is drawn for laboratory studies and x-ray films are ordered. In a short while the patient tells the nurse she is tired of waiting and is going home. What is the first and most important step for the nurse to take in this AMA situation?

0   A. Determine the patient's competency to decide refusal
0   B. Assist the patient in understanding the risks involved in leaving
0   C. Have the patient sign the AMA form on her way out
0   D. Try to convince the patient to stay

Patient Transfer

11. A 21-year-old uninsured paranoid schizophrenic patient who has been deeply depressed has attempted suicide. She is brought to the community hospital emergency department with a large laceration on the right side of her neck and one on her left upper arm. She has some active bleeding from the arm, which is controlled with a pressure bandage. The emergency department physician asks the nurse to arrange a transfer to the county hospital because they have emergency psychiatric services available. Before transport, the most important thing the nurse should ensure is that the:

0   A. Patient consents to the transfer
0   B. Receiving hospital agrees to the transfer
0   C. Reason for the transfer is clear and justifiable
0   D. Patient is stabilized prior to the transfer and deemed safe for transport

ANSWERS

1. **B. Analysis.** Based on the patient's history and assessment, he is at great risk for falling and causing physical injury to himself.[2,3]
2. **A. Intervention.** Side rails up and locked in place, along with a jacket restraint device, are needed to prevent possible falls.[2,3]
3. **A. Analysis.** Negligence, to be alleged and proved in court, must consist of four elements: (1) duty (accepting responsibility for care and then being obligated to provide acceptable care), (2) breech of duty (not providing care according to accepted standards), (3) damage or injury (damage must have occurred), and (4) proximate cause (a cause-and-effect relationship between damage and breech of duty must exist). In

this case the nurse had a duty to protect this patient with an altered mental status from harm and injury. She neither put up the side rail nor restrained the patient. The damage (fractured hip and wrist) resulted because of this negligence, although it was unintentional on the part of the nurse.[2,3]

4. **D. Intervention.** Expression of feelings is most essential at this time.[2,3]

5. **C. Intervention.** CISD offers immediate debriefing to individuals by uninvolved, objective persons who are trained in this area. CISD assists in dealing with immediate emotional reactions to specific critical incidents so that individuals become more prepared to cope effectively with situations. It may also help prevent delayed stress or emotional reactions related to the incident. CISD also offers referral to those who appear to exhibit ineffective coping behaviors.[2,3]

6. **D. Intervention.** JCAHO requires documented proof of *A, B,* and *C.* Orientation on beginning employment *only* is unsatisfactory, because ongoing education and annual competency skills testing are mandatory as well.[2,4]

7. **A. Intervention.** The rights of human subjects must be a priority in research endeavors. If the research protocol has outlined that a consent is to be signed, that policy must be adhered to. The role of the emergency department nurse in conjunction with research endeavors is often one of ensuring patient safety.[3]

8. **A. Intervention.** If a minor is brought to the emergency department by anyone other than the parents, all attempts must be made to contact the parents before treatment is rendered unless a life-threatening situation exists.[2]

9. **C. Intervention.** The first priority should be safety for all parties involved in providing emergency care.[1-4]

10. **A. Intervention.** The patient's competency to leave against medical advice must be determined. A competent, conscious patient has the right to refuse treatment if he or she understands the consequences of refusal. This should be confirmed by a signature on the AMA form. The patient's chart should include documentation that the risks and/or consequences of leaving against medical advice were explained.[2]

11. **D. Intervention.** While all of these steps must be taken, the most important is the safety of the patient. The COBRA law requires that any hospital receiving Medicare funds evaluate all emergency patients to determine whether an emergency condition exists. If it does, the hospital must provide immediate and stabilizing care before a transfer is considered.[5,6]

REFERENCES

1. Frank I: *Managing emergency nursing services,* Rockville, Md, 1989, Aspen.
2. Northrop CE, Kelly ME: *Legal issues in nursing,* St Louis, 1987, Mosby–Year Book.
3. Rae R et al: *Emergency nursing core curriculum,* ed 3, Philadelphia, 1987, WB Saunders.
4. Joint Commission on the Accreditation of Hospitals and Health Care Organizations: *Accreditation manual for hospitals, emergency services,* Chicago, 1990, The Commission.
5. Kitt S: Interfacility transfer. In Kitt S, Kaiser J, editors: *Emergency nursing: a physiologic and clinical perspective,* Philadephia, 1990, WB Saunders.
6. Harrahill M, Bartkus E: Preparing the trauma patient for transfer, *JEN* 9(4):234, 1983.

ADDITIONAL READINGS

Buschiazzo L: *The Handbook of emergency nursing management.* Rockville, Md, 1987, Aspen.

Emergency Department Nurses Association (EDMA): *Standards of emergency nursing practice,* St Louis, 1983, Mosby–Year Book.

Lack R: Quality assurance in the emergency department. In Kitt S, Kaiser J, editors: *Emergency nursing: a physiologic and clinical perspective,* Philadelphia, 1990, WB Saunders.

Punch L: Hospital must restructure emergency charges to retain patient case, *Mod Health* 10:122, 1989.

Schulmerich SC: Developing a patient classification system for the emergency department, *JEN* 10:298-305, 1989.

Southard PA: COBRA legislation: complying with emergency department provisions, *JEN* 156(1):23-25, 1989.

Vestal KW: Marketing concepts for the emergency department, *JEN* 9:290-293, 1989.

Vestal KW: Promoting excellence in the emergency department, *JEN* 10:290-293, 1989.

Young D, White B: Fiscal considerations in a competitive environment. In Kitt S, Kaiser J, editors: *Emergency nursing: a physiologic and clinical perspective,* Philadelphia, 1990, WB Saunders.

Chapter 25

Disaster Preparedness and Management

REVIEW OUTLINE

I. General overview
   A. Disaster: defined as any patient-generating incident that results in overload of either existing personnel or existing supplies and equipment, or any patient-generating incident that occurs in a situation wherein resources for backup of staff and equipment are not available in a reasonable amount of time.[1]
   B. Categories of disaster
      1. Natural: violence of nature
      2. Man-made: human error
   C. Effects of disasters
      1. Loss of life
      2. Physical injuries
      3. Psychological trauma
      4. Property damage
      5. Environmental destruction
   D. Joint Commission on Accreditation of Health Organizations (JCAHO) requirements: hospital must devise, implement, and practice (twice a year) a hospital-wide disaster plan
   E. Key components of a disaster plan
      1. Patient care
         a. Receiving, triaging, distributing
         b. Proper use of resources and/or facility
         c. Documenting care
         d. Evaluating care
      2. Communication

a. Internal
b. External
c. News media
d. Command post
3. Resources
    a. Personnel
    b. Supplies
    c. Security
    d. Coordination
    e. Hospital resources
    f. Community resources
4. Security, safety
    a. Traffic control
    b. Controlled access to department
5. Coordination
    a. Local, state, federal
    b. Intradepartmental, interdepartmental
6. Documentation
    a. Medical record
    b. Disaster tag
    c. Paper flow
F. Six stages of disaster
    1. Warning
    2. Impact
    3. Inventory
    4. Rescue
    5. Remedy
    6. Recovery
G. Disaster triage
    1. In the field
    2. In the emergency department
II. Nursing role in disaster management
   A. Development of the plan
       1. Key components (see section I, E)
       2. Practice, evaluate, revise
   B. Implementation of the plan
   C. Command post
       1. Communications: internal, external
       2. Dealing with news media
       3. Hospital/departmental command post

INTRODUCTION

A disaster is defined as any patient-generating incident that results in overload of either existing personnel or existing supplies and equipment, or any patient-generating incident that occurs in a situation wherein resources for backup of staff and equipment are not available in a reasonable amount of time.[1]

There are two categories of disasters: natural and man-made. Natural disasters are incidents of violence of nature, such as a tornado, hurricane, earthquake, or epidemic. Man-made disasters are incidents of human error such as fire, explosion, nuclear incidents, or transportation accidents.[2] Natural and man-made disasters present a serious threat to the health and welfare of all people throughout the world.

Hospitals are required by the JCAHO to prepare for disaster situations. The JCAHO requires hospitals to devise, implement, and practice (twice a year) a hospital-wide disaster plan and a specific emergency department disaster plan. The emergency department plan must include detailed guidelines that collaboratively interface with both the hospital and the community plans. Key components of disaster plans include patient care, communication, resources, safety or security, coordination, and documentation.

Greater risks for disaster situations exist in the world today. Emergency department personnel must be familiar with their disaster plan and know their role in executing the plan when needed. They also need to understand the stages of a disaster so that they can better understand what has happened to patients prior to their arrival in the emergency department and what they will likely experience after discharge. The stages of a disaster are warning, impact, inventory, rescue, remedy, and recovery.

The role of the emergency department nurse in disaster management involves many areas: development and practice of the plan, implementation of the plan, development of a command post to serve as a communication link with the hospital and external environment, triage activities, secondary triage, stabilization, and critical incident stress debriefing. Emergency nurses are a "natural" for disaster management because of their rapid assessment and triage skills, crisis management abilities, and linkages with community resource persons.

Chemical and Radiation Disasters

Of specific concern is knowing how to handle both chemical and radiation disaster situations. Knowing that staff members have familiarity with the departmental disaster plan and are aware of their role in the plan is important. Donning the proper attire, using the proper procedures, and evaluating the disaster drills in which one participates are all important to the efficient functioning of the staff during a real situation. Practice helps keep the staff and patients safe and makes for a smoother operation when a real disaster occurs.

The emergency department plan must provide for the efficient management of incoming casualties and must include charge nurse responsibilities, disposition of patients currently in the department, preparation of the triage site, patient flow, extent of initial and ongoing treatment, alternate patient care areas, and staffing and supply needs.

Sanford[3] describes the eight principles of disaster management: preventing the occurrence of a disaster, minimizing the number of casualties, rescuing, providing first aid, evacuating the injured, providing definitive care, facilitating reconstruction, and recovery.[4] Whether in the prehospital care arena or in the emergency department, the emergency nurse is best prepared to handle disaster situations. It is important, however, for the nurse to be aware of the differences in triage priorities "in the field" versus in the emergency department.

A comprehensive disaster system incorporates the community, the hospital, the emergency department, and the local, state, and federal domain. Disaster preparedness requires careful planning, frequent practice, critiques, and ongoing revision. The emergency department nurse must be knowledgeable about these disaster systems and be in a state of readiness to quickly implement and execute the plan.

REVIEW QUESTIONS
Mass Casualty Disaster

There has been an explosion at a chemical plant in an inner-city area. Employees, persons passing by in cars, and people in nearby houses and buildings have also been injured. The number of injuries is unknown. The emergency nurse has been called to assist with field triage and on arrival finds the following victims:

No. 1: *28-year-old man in acute respiratory distress who is cyanotic and diaphoretic. Vital signs are blood pressure, 70/40; pulse, 140; and respiratory rate, 40 with labored respirations. There is bruising on the left side of the chest.*

No. 2: *64-year-old man in cardiac arrest with dilated and fixed pupils. There is no pulse or respirations. There are no physical signs of injury.*

No. 3: *30-year-old pregnant woman who is full term and in active labor with contractions every 5 minutes. This is her fourth child. She is upset and crying. There are no physical signs of injury.*

No. 4: *35-year-old woman with head, face, and leg lacerations with bleeding. She is incoherent. Her vital signs are blood pressure, 96/60; pulse, 110; and respiratory rate, 30.*

No. 5: *60-year-old man with a head laceration who is unresponsive to verbal or painful stimuli. Vital signs are blood pressure, 100/70; pulse, 96; and respiratory rate, 24.*

1. Which patient should be cared for *first?*
   0 A. Patient No. 1
   0 B. Patient No. 2
   0 C. Patient No. 3
   0 D. Patient No. 4

2. The most obvious nursing diagnosis for patient No. 1 in this scenario is:
   0 A. Airway clearance, ineffective
   0 B. Tissue perfusion, altered
   0 C. Gas exchange, impaired
   0 D. Cardiac output, decreased

3. Which patient in this scenario should receive *last* priority for treatment?
   0   A. Patient No. 2
   0   B. Patient No. 3
   0   C. Patient No. 4
   0   D. Patient No. 5

Internal Disasters

4. The nurse who enters an internal disaster scene should begin an evaluation to control the disaster. The first and foremost step for the emergency nurse to take is to:
   0   A. Take photographs of the situation
   0   B. Tell everyone else to stand back while the nurse cares for the victims
   0   C. Assess and assure the safety of the area
   0   D. Notify the National Disaster Management Services (NDMS)

Radiation Disasters

5. The emergency nurse receives a patient who has been exposed to radiation into the decontamination room. The largest part of the decontamination procedure is accomplished by:
   0   A. Removing the patient's clothing
   0   B. Washing the patient with soap and water
   0   C. Washing the patient with water only
   0   D. Using a specific antidote for the contaminant

6. Two major principles nurses should employ in caring for individuals in a radiation accident/hazardous materials incident include (select two answers):
   0   A. Preventing further exposure
   0   B. Providing appropriate treatment immediately
   0   C. Notifying the patient's family
   0   D. Calling the state health and safety regulatory agency immediately

7. The emergency department receives a critically injured contaminated victim. The first priority of the emergency department nurse should be to:
   0   A. Start radiation exposure evaluation
   0   B. Control contamination to a specific area

   0   C. Resuscitate and stabilize the victim
   0   D. Decontaminate the victim

8. Radiation exposure evaluation begins with all of the following *except:*
   0   A. Nausea and vomiting, and/or anorexia
   0   B. Erythema
   0   C. Baseline complete blood cell counts
   0   D. Visual disturbances or cataracts

9. Personnel resuscitating and decontaminating a radiation-exposed patient should wear all of the following *except:*
   0   A. A scrub suit
   0   B. Headgear and masks
   0   C. Double-latex gloves
   0   D. A rad meter (dosimeter)

Disaster Communication

10. The most important aspect of maintaining adequate communications during a disaster is to have a(n):
   0   A. Effective charge nurse
   0   B. Efficiently functioning command post
   0   C. Direct line to the news media to give frequent updates
   0   D. Video camera to tape the event

11. Following a disaster event, the staff may need to deal with their feelings about the situation and the patients they cared for. This could best be accomplished by:
   0   A. Calling the chaplain to come to the emergency department
   0   B. Asking the staff to talk openly in a group session with the nurse manager as the facilitator
   0   C. Calling the critical incident stress debriefing (CISD) team
   0   D. Asking a physician to prescribe sleeping medication for all personnel who request it

12. The most important tool to have in the emergency department to serve as a first line of defense for disasters is a(n):
   0   A. Well-defined disaster plan
   0   B. A medical director who has disaster medicine experience
   0   C. Red Cross nurse on staff
   0   D. Alarm system that connects to the local fire department

ANSWERS

1. **A. Assessment.** Always remember the airway, breathing, circulation rule and that field triage is geared toward saving the greatest number of lives using the simplest measures possible. Triage in the emergency department is focused on doing the greatest good for the greatest number. For patient No. 1, an airway needs to be established or cleared; the patient then needs to be transported to the emergency department.[2,3,5,6]

2. **A. Analysis.** The patient's airway is not patent. The airway must be opened so that breathing and circulation issues can be further assessed.[7]

3. **A. Assessment.** The life of this patient could not be saved "simply" or in a short period of time. Other patients whose lives might be saved would have to wait if this patient were dealt with first.[2,3,5,6]

4. **C. Intervention.** The nurse who goes to a disaster situation should do a three-step evaluation of (1) the safety of the area, (2) the organization of the disaster system, and (3) the provision of the most appropriate patient care.[2,3,5,6]

5. **A. Intervention.** Ninety to ninety-five percent of the decontamination procedure is accomplished by removing the patient's clothing. The clothing is placed in bags, tagged, and removed to a remote section of the contaminated area to be disposed of later by qualified personnel. The remaining decontamination is accomplished by washing the patient with soap and water.[8]

6. **A, B. Intervention.**[8]

7. **C. Intervention.** While all the answers are principles to follow in the care of injured contaminated patients, the first priority is to resuscitate and stabilize the victim. The order of priority after that is *D, B, A*.[8]

8. **D. Assessment.** Visual disturbances are not usually a primary complaint of radiation-exposed patients.[8]

9. **A. Intervention.** A scrub suit would not be appropriate dress if the emergency nurse were going to participate in the decontamination of a patient who had been exposed to radiation. A disposable full body suit should be worn.

10. **B. Intervention.** The command post is the vital link between the field and the participating hospital and serves as a "command central" for communications.[6]

11. **C. Intervention.** The debriefing team is best prepared to handle this situation. Team members remain objective and are most helpful to the staff, enabling them to discuss their feelings and providing a tool to prevent and alleviate symptoms created by the event. This offers immediate crisis intervention, helping the staff to return to their precrisis level of functioning.[9]

12. **A. Evaluation.** A well-defined disaster plan that has been practiced and critiqued will provide emergency nurses with guidelines for dealing with real disaster situations.[6]

REFERENCES

1. Simoneau JK: Disaster management. In Sheehy SB, Barber J: *Emergency nursing: principles and practice,* ed 2, St Louis, 1985, Mosby–Year Book.
2. Parker JG: Disaster planning. In Parker JG, editor: *Emergency nursing: a guide to comprehensive care,* New York, 1984, John Wiley & Sons.
3. Sanford JP: Civilian disasters and disaster planning. In Burkle S, Sanner P, Wolcott B, editors: *Disaster medicine,* New York, 1984, Medical Examination Publishing.
4. Richtsmeier JL, Miller JR: Psychological aspects to disaster situations. In Garcia LM, editor: *Disaster nursing: planning, assessment, and intervention,* Rockville, Md, 1985, Aspen.
5. Burkle S, Sanner P, Wolcott B, editors: *Disaster medicine,* New York, 1984, Medical Examination Publishing.
6. Garcia LM: *Disaster nursing: planning, assessment, and intervention,* Rockville, Md, 1985, Aspen.
7. Rea R et al: *Nursing core curriculum,* ed 3, Philadelphia, 1987, WB Saunders.
8. Bonet A: Mass casualty management. In Kitt S, Kaiser, J, editors: *Emergency nursing: a physiologic and clinical perspective,* Philadelphia, 1990, WB Saunders.
9. Mitchell JT: When disaster strikes . . . the CISD process, *J Emerg Med Serv* 8(30):6, 1983.

ADDITIONAL READINGS

Lanros N: *Assessment and intervention in emergency nursing,* ed 2, Bowie, Md, 1983, Robert J Brady.
National Council on Radiation Protection and Measurements: *Management of persons accidentally contaminated with radionuclides,* Report No 65, Bethesda, Md, 1985, US Government Printing Office.
Rubin J: Critical incident stress debriefing: helping the helpers, *JEN* 16(4):255-258, 1990.
Sheehy SB, Barber J: *Emergency nursing: principles and practice,* ed 2, St Louis, 1985, Mosby–Year Book.
Walsh M: *Accident and emergency nursing: a new approach,* ed 2, Oxford, United Kingdom, 1990, Heinemann Medical.

Index _____